HYPOGLYCEMIA: Fact or Fad?

What You Should Know about Low Blood Sugar

LYNN J. BENNION, M.D.

CONSUMERS UNION
Mount Vernon, New York

This special Consumers Union edition of *Hypoglycemia: Fact or Fad?*
has been published by arrangement with Crown Publishers, Inc.

Library of Congress Cataloging in Publication Data
Bennion, Lynn J.
Hypoglycemia: fact or fad?
Glossary: p. 163
Includes index.
1. Hypoglycemia I. Title.
RC662.2.B46 1983 616.4'66 83–10060
ISBN: 0-89043-135-3

Consumers Union edition
First printing, April, 1986

Hypoglycemia: Fact or Fad? is a Consumer Reports Book published by Consumers Union, the nonprofit organization that publishes *Consumer Reports,* the monthly magazine of test reports, product Ratings, and buying guidance. Established in 1936, Consumers Union is chartered under the Not-For-Profit Corporation Law of the State of New York.

The purposes of Consumers Union, as stated in its charter, are to provide consumers with information and counsel on consumer goods and services, to give information on all matters relating to the expenditure of the family income, and to initiate and to cooperate with individual and group efforts seeking to create and maintain decent living standards.

Consumers Union derives its income solely from the sale of *Consumer Reports* and other publications. In addition, expenses of occasional public service efforts may be met, in part, by nonrestrictive, noncommercial contributions, grants, and fees. Consumers Union accepts no advertising or product samples and is not beholden in any way to any commercial interest. Its Ratings and reports are solely for the use of the readers of its publications. Neither the Ratings nor the reports nor any Consumers Union publications, including this book, may be used in advertising or for any commercial purpose. Consumers Union will take all steps open to it to prevent such uses of its material, its name, or the name of *Consumer Reports*.

Manufactured in the United States of America

To my wife
No Aladdin
ever had
a better Genie

Read not to contradict, nor to believe,
but to weigh and consider.

—FRANCIS BACON, *Of Studies*, 1597

Foreword to the Consumers Union Edition

Fatigue, insomnia, irritability, weakness, depression, mood swings, and a host of other common complaints most people feel at one time or another. Since the early fifties, following the publication of *Body, Mind, and Sugar* by Drs. Abrahamson and Pezet, these symptoms have been ascribed by food faddists, health "promoters," and a few physicians to one cause—low blood sugar. Treatments offered for this disorder have ranged from expensive injections of an extract made from the adrenal glands of hogs and cows to megadoses of vitamins, minerals, brewer's yeast, and other nostrums. Low blood sugar—technically called hypoglycemia—has become a subject of widespread misunderstanding — no thanks to misinformation disseminated by the now-defunct Hypoglycemia Foundation and by the popular press. The frequency of this disorder has also been exaggerated by medical misdiagnosis and outright quackery. With the publication of this special edition of *Hypoglycemia: Fact or Fad?* we seek to provide consumers with clear, authoritative information about low blood sugar.

As early as 1971, *Consumer Reports* published an article titled "Low Blood Sugar: Fact and Fiction," which called attention to flaws inherent in the treatment rationale of low blood sugar proponents. The article concluded that injections of adrenal cortex extract (ACE) had no place in the treatment of the disorder. Eventually, the U.S. Food and Drug Administration ordered ACE off the market, stating in 1977: "There is no evidence it is effective in treating burns, low blood sugar, alcohol or drug addiction, or any other disease."

Consumers Union "blew the whistle" on the faulty reasoning behind the claims that hypoglycemia was responsible for the multitude of symptoms attributed to it. CU also called attention to the difference between organic and functional hypoglycemia, including the relative infrequency of the disorder. Such information was well-known to the medical profession, which to that point had done little to offset the propaganda of the Hypoglycemia Foundation and those few physicians who supported it.

It was not until 1973 that CU found official medical backing in its stand. In that year, the American Diabetes Association, the American Medical Association, and the Endocrine Society issued a joint statement echoing our position. The organizations asserted that the "majority of people" experiencing sweating, shakiness, trembling, anxiety, fast heart action, hunger sensations, brief feelings of weakness, and occasionally seizures and coma, "do not have hypoglycemia."

The withdrawal of adrenal cortex extract from the market and statements from recognized professional organizations trimmed the sails of the quacks somewhat, but unfortunately, have not entirely stemmed the tide of misinformation that continues to abound around this uncommon disorder. People are still being misdiagnosed as being hypoglycemic and are given lists of foods to avoid and told to maintain a schedule of small, frequent daily meals. In this book, Dr. Lynn J. Bennion, a specialist in endocrinology and human metabolism, offers a clear perspective for doctors and medical consumers alike. He defines the disorder, describes its symptoms, details its causes in children and adults, and gives practical advice on treatment.

Also, Dr. Bennion offers a very sensible critique of the five-hour oral glucose tolerance test (OGTT)—a test that is still widely used to diagnose hypoglycemia. He concludes that the OGTT is not reliable and may even be misleading. This information may spare you, family members, friends, and acquaintances from the unnecessary expense and discomfort of this procedure.

As is always the case when we publish an edition of a book not of our own creation, the information and advice contained herein are that of the author, not of Consumers Union.

—The Editors of Consumer Reports Books

Contents

Acknowledgments

Many teachers and patients provided ideas, instruction, and examples essential to this book. Peter S. Stevens and Helene Schellenberg Barnhart deserve special thanks for deft and gentle surgery on several chapters. I appreciate also the encouragement of Lota and Walter V. Davidson, Jr., and other friends and family members.

Preface

This book began in a doctor's office. Its moment of conception came as I heard myself repeat to a patient the same facts I had just explained to someone else a few hours earlier. Both patients had been referred to me because of low blood sugar, or hypoglycemia. Each had distressing symptoms, and in each the distress was compounded by confusion and misunderstanding. Those patients, like so many others who have hypoglycemia, or who suspect they have it, needed a straightforward explanation of the facts about low blood sugar.

I ought to tape-record this speech, I thought, as I reviewed the same material with each individual. Or perhaps a booklet in the waiting room would help these people. I settled on the idea of a booklet, but as pen met paper, important points needed amplification through actual case histories, and this book came into being.

I wrote the book for the lay public—especially for those who have been told or suspect they have hypoglycemia, or who believe someone dear to them has it. While patients might introduce the book to their family physicians, the material is directed more to the patient than to the doctor. Physicians, however, might profitably refer their patients to the book in order to clear up some of the widespread confusion that exists on the subject.

I wish to caution the reader that no book can substitute for a sympathetic and well-informed physician. This is not a do-it-yourself guidebook to self-diagnosis or a manual of home health care. It will, however, enable you to understand blood sugar, grasp why it is important, see how the human body normally regulates it, and learn what can go wrong to result in hypoglycemia. That understanding will permit you, in cooperation with a physician, to approach intelligently the problems associated with hypoglycemia, and to solve them successfully in your own particular case.

Introduction

Ernest[1] came to my office concerned about hypoglycemia. This 19-year-old man appeared healthy, bright, and energetic. He worked days as assistant manager of a grocery store and attended college classes at night.

A year earlier Ernest had sought help from his family doctor because of headaches and fatigue. He and his doctor had discussed his symptoms in detail, including a light-headed, lethargic feeling that seemed to follow the intake of certain foods. Other symptoms, such as inability to concentrate and difficulty coping with stress, had begun to cripple his progress at work and school and his social life.

Ernest's doctor diagnosed his case as hypoglycemia, and explained that all of his symptoms stemmed from that one basic problem.

The doctor prescribed a special diet, restricted in sugars and carbohydrates and many of the foods this young man was accustomed to eating. Ernest followed the diet faithfully and felt better at first. But then his symptoms returned. He therefore adhered more strictly to the diet, with the consequent loss of 15 pounds. He became increasingly exhausted, intolerant of various foods, and unable to function well as a student or employee.

The final straw came when his fiancée broke off their engagement because of his increasing disabilities. Ernest decided to seek the help of a specialist in endocrinology and metabolism. Since

[1] Throughout the book, all personal names and identifying details have been changed.

my last name starts with B and was therefore listed first in the Yellow Pages for that specialty, he came to my office.

It turned out that Ernest did not have hypoglycemia at all, though many of his symptoms were compatible with that diagnosis. The rest of his story is recounted later in this book, but the point to be made here is that while hypoglycemia is fairly common, mistaken ideas about it are even more common. Like many other people, Ernest and his physician held misconceptions about hypoglycemia derived from unscientific misinformation prevalent in the popular media. Those misconceptions prevent proper diagnosis and treatment of people with hypoglycemia. They also obstruct intelligent treatment of many other people, like Ernest, whose symptoms resemble those of hypoglycemia but actually arise from other problems.

Hypoglycemia has become one of the most discussed but least understood topics in modern medicine. So popular is the diagnosis that many people, including some doctors, see it as a serious epidemic. Others call hypoglycemia a fad, and claim that the real epidemic is one of misunderstanding and misdiagnosis. With this in mind, I ask the reader to remember: "It ain't what you don't know that makes you ignorant; it's what you know that ain't so!" Some of what you think you know about hypoglycemia may not be true, so please read with an open mind. For my part, I'll try to adhere to the guideline of the famous criminal investigator Sergeant Friday: "Just the facts, ma'am."

So many different theories and explanations of hypoglycemia have been put forward that it would take several volumes to explain and refute each one in detail. Fiction and falsehood come in infinite variety. Fortunately, however, the facts are fairly simple. This book will therefore focus on *what is known* about blood sugar, its normal regulation in the human body, and what can go wrong to result in hypoglycemia. It will not seek to acquaint the reader with the details of the many fanciful theories and misunderstandings that have been popular for too long.

This book does not contain "the final word" about blood glucose metabolism. Scientific knowledge is continually expanding with new research, and in the future new discoveries will no doubt improve our understanding of the subject.

Reliable research is likely to be published first in carefully edited scientific journals, such as the *Journal of Clinical Investigation,* the

Journal of Clinical Endocrinology and Metabolism, or the *New England Journal of Medicine,* rather than in the *National Enquirer.* In scientific journals, articles are scrutinized by experts prior to publication, and the experimental methods that were used to find the facts and form the conclusions are printed in detail. Other scientists can then repeat the experiment and check the conclusions. While not foolproof, this system allows errors to be detected and corrected, and provides firm footing for the promotion of health and the practice of medicine. These checks and balances of science have not been applied to much of what has masqueraded in the popular media as expert advice about hypoglycemia.

Misunderstanding about hypoglycemia extends even to the meaning of the word itself. Our first chapter, therefore, explains what hypoglycemia is and what it is not.

1

What Is Hypoglycemia?

To begin our understanding of hypoglycemia, let's break the word down. *Hypo* means "low." *Glyc* refers to "glucose," the chemical form of sugar found in the bloodstream. *Emia* means "in the blood." Putting the parts together, we have the word *hypoglycemia,* which means "low blood sugar."

Sugar, or glucose, travels in the bloodstream to all parts of the body. After it leaves the bloodstream and enters the cells that make up the tissues of the body, glucose serves as fuel for the body's tissues. It is an energy source.

When someone doesn't have enough glucose in the bloodstream to satisfy the energy needs of the body for normal function, the condition of hypoglycemia exists. Simply defined, hypoglycemia means that the level of blood glucose is too low to meet the immediate energy needs of body tissues.

When there is not enough gasoline in the tank of your car, your car is useless. It can't function. So it is with your body. Although your body may contain plenty of stored energy in the form of fat, or other potential energy sources such as protein, without enough glucose immediately available in the bloodstream, certain tissues cease to function properly.

The tissues of the nervous system—brain, spinal cord, and nerves—depend on glucose as an energy source. Many other tissues, such as muscles, can get along well using fats as an energy source, but *the brain must have glucose*. During prolonged starvation, the brain can adjust to use *ketones* (a breakdown product of fat) to satisfy part of its energy needs. However, the brain always needs a certain minimal supply of glucose to function normally.

Hypoglycemia is not the only cause of malfunction of tissues such as the brain that depend on glucose for energy. The condition called *hypoxemia*, meaning "low blood oxygen," can act much the same as hypoglycemia, since the body must have oxygen to derive energy from the glucose.

Again using our gasoline analogy, an automobile requires air to mix with the gasoline in order to achieve combustion and produce power. Lack of air, lack of gasoline, or lack of electrical spark can all produce the same frustrating situation—a car that won't start. Likewise, lack of glucose (hypoglycemia), lack of oxygen (hypoxemia), and lack of other necessary ingredients, such as phosphate (hypophosphatemia), can produce a lack of energy and malfunction of body tissues.

Hypoglycemia, then, is not any particular set of symptoms, and the symptoms we associate with it are not necessarily unique to that condition. Don't jump to the conclusion that you have hypoglycemia because you crave sweets or get a sick, dizzy feeling after eating rich chocolate cake. If your heart races and your palms sweat during a sales presentation or public speech, don't be too hasty to conclude that something is wrong with your blood sugar. To lay all the blame for fatigue, irritability, or hunger on hypoglycemia is like claiming that every time your car won't start it's out of gasoline.

In the same way that many different causes produce a car that won't run, many different causes produce symptoms popularly attributed to hypoglycemia. Hypoglycemia is not a "nervous condition" or any other sort of condition describable by a unique set of symptoms.

Since the symptoms of hypoglycemia are *not specific* for that condition but can be caused as well by entirely different problems, you cannot make the diagnosis of hypoglycemia solely on the basis of your symptoms. You may suspect you have hypoglycemia on the basis of your symptoms, but whether they really arise from hypoglycemia depends on the actual level of your blood sugar.

A personal note, although not about hypoglycemia, should clarify this point.

I have always had such a pale complexion that my mother was sure I was *anemic.* This prompted her to feed me lots of liver, a previously popular remedy for anemia. After many excruciating meals of liver, my complexion remained sallow. Perhaps, my mother thought, I needed iron pills, since everyone knows that anemia means your blood count is low, and that iron helps build your blood. Thus two iron pills appeared each morning on my breakfast plate. Still the sun didn't rise in my cheeks. Pale as moonlight, I arrived in the kitchen each morning for breakfast to find the two iron pills joined by several brewer's yeast tablets and a long green multivitamin pill that made me burp until noon. As a result of all this nutrition, I grew to be six inches taller than my parents, but my complexion stayed pale.

Anemia, which is a shortage of red blood cells, or hemoglobin, in the bloodstream, can indeed make you pale. On the other hand, there are other causes of a pasty complexion, such as spending too much time indoors or having Scandinavian ancestors. Just a pale complexion doesn't prove you have anemia.

If you want to find out whether someone is anemic, you have to put a needle into his or her vein and draw blood for a laboratory test: a blood hemoglobin level. When this test was finally applied to me, it turned out I wasn't anemic after all. The hemoglobin level was normal. The pallid complexion had been due to something else—probably my ancestry or my habit of spending too much time indoors reading. Getting outside and gardening in the sun does more for my complexion than a truckload of little liver pills.

Now, the same logic applies to hypoglycemia. Although a person may have symptoms consistent with hypoglycemia, such as fatigue or confusion, you have to *measure* the sugar content of the blood before you can logically conclude that low blood sugar is the culprit. Many conditions may cause symptoms identical to those of hypoglycemia, but treatments aimed at raising the blood sugar should be reserved for those people whose blood sugar has been shown to be *measurably* low.

I want to return now to the analogy of anemia to make another important point. Suppose a person really *is* anemic. Would lots of liver and iron pills be an intelligent treatment? Maybe. Maybe not. It depends on *why* the person is anemic.

Anemia is not a disease. It is a low blood hemoglobin level. If someone is anemic, there is something wrong that is causing the hemoglobin level to be low. The first step is not a trial of liver and iron therapy. The intelligent first step is to figure out *why* the person has anemia. Malaria might be the cause of the anemia, or hookworms in the intestine, or a bleeding ulcer, or a cancer of the rectum. Or in a child it might be lead poisoning from chewing on lead paint on the windowsill.

The proper treatment for anemia depends on what is causing it. In one case the remedy might be drugs to cure hookworms, but in another it might be rectal surgery to remove a cancer, or medications to heal an ulcer. For the child it might be a coat of lead-free latex paint on the window ledge.

The point is that anemia is not in itself a disease or an indication for a specific form of treatment. It is an abnormality detected in a blood test. It *demands* that a more specific diagnosis be made so that intelligent treatment can be given.

So it is with low blood sugar. Hypoglycemia is not in itself a disease or an indication for a specific form of treatment. It is an abnormality detected in a blood test. It *demands* that a more specific diagnosis be made so that intelligent treatment can be given.

Unfortunately, the popular myths about hypoglycemia treat it as if it were a single disease. This misconception leads directly to the notion that there is a single treatment for it. A variety of remedies have been prescribed for this "disease," but none of them are appropriate until a more specific diagnosis has been made. The most popular remedy has been a diet low in carbohydrates and high in protein, taken in frequent small feedings. This kind of diet is indeed helpful in treating one of the causes of hypoglycemia. To prescribe the diet to everyone with hypoglycemia makes no more sense than feeding liver or hookworm pills to everyone with anemia.

To make matters worse, many people have been pronounced hypoglycemic without proof that their blood sugar levels are actually lower than normal. Like a loving mother who diagnosed anemia on the basis of a pale complexion, many well-intentioned physicians have diagnosed hypoglycemia solely on the basis of symptoms. That was the mistake Ernest's[1] doctor made. Still other practitioners have been misinformed—by supposedly authoritative sources—about what levels of blood glucose are

[1] **See Introduction.**

normal and what are abnormal. Some physicians become so frustrated that they refuse to believe hypoglycemia exists, and refuse to see or treat patients who think they may have it. We'll cover the issues of how to diagnose hypoglycemia, and how to find its cause, in later chapters of this book. Before leaving this chapter, however, the reader should understand clearly that hypoglycemia does exist, and that when it exists there is a reason for it.

The following case illustrates how, by probing deeper into the causes of hypoglycemia, a physician can make a specific diagnosis and give appropriate therapy.

Enrique Engelhardt came to the emergency room of Massachusetts General Hospital feeling weak and dizzy. His back hurt, he couldn't eat without vomiting, and when he tried to stand up he almost passed out. The resident physician in the emergency room called a new intern—fresh out of medical school—and told him, "I've got a patient down here for you by the name of Engelhardt. He has low blood sugar, low blood pressure, low blood sodium, and low body temperature. He is being admitted on your service."

When the intern examined Mr. Engelhardt he learned that three weeks earlier the man had been operated on for clogging within the blood vessels of his legs. After the operation there had been problems with infections. Then blood clots had lodged in Mr. Engelhardt's lungs. Powerful drugs were therefore given to prevent clotting.

Mr. Engelhardt appeared weak and thin. His rectal temperature was only 96.2 degrees (normal is about 99). His blood pressure was below normal as he lay flat in bed, but as soon as he sat up it would fall much lower—so low that he would almost pass out. The blood chemistries showed a glucose level of 20 (definitely low) and a sodium level of 118 (normal is about 140). He was in obvious pain and distress and was too sick to eat.

The intern noticed another abnormality in the laboratory tests, an excessive number of eosinophil cells in the blood—and that triggered his recollection that when the adrenal glands aren't working the eosinophil cell count rises, and the blood pressure, blood sodium, and blood glucose may fall to abnormally low levels.

A budding endocrinologist, the intern ordered blood and urine tests necessary to determine whether Mr. Engelhardt's adrenal glands were working. Since a patient can go into shock and die if adrenal glands aren't working, the intern treated Mr. Engelhardt with a large intravenous dose of adrenal-gland hormone, and Enrique started to feel better. Within a few hours his appetite returned, and his blood pressure, blood sodium, and blood sugar all came back to normal.

The blood and urine tests later showed conclusively that this intern's hunch had been right: Mr. Engelhardt's adrenal glands had been destroyed and weren't making their essential hormones. Those hormones, in the form of hydrocortisone, had to be given daily to prevent a return of the low blood glucose, low blood pressure, and other manifestations of adrenal-gland failure. As long as he took his hydrocortisone, Mr. Engelhardt felt fine, but when he skipped it, his symptoms of nausea, weakness, and dizziness returned.

Mr. Engelhardt did have hypoglycemia: His blood glucose was abnormally low. But hypoglycemia was not his disease; it was a manifestation of his disease. The low blood sugar was simply a clue that something was wrong. His disease was adrenal-gland failure, caused in all likelihood by bleeding into the adrenal glands, destroying them and thereby cutting off the body's supply of adrenal-gland hormones. This is a rare side effect of taking too much of the medicine prescribed to counteract the blood clots in his lungs.

For treatment Mr. Engelhardt needed replacement of those missing adrenal hormones, either by injection or by pills. A low-carbohydrate, high-protein, frequent-small-feeding diet will not take care of adrenal-gland failure. Hydrocortisone will. A diagnosis more specific than hypoglycemia led to a specific, rational, and helpful treatment.

Mr. Engelhardt's case is unusually dramatic, but it illustrates a fact common to all cases of hypoglycemia: *If* the blood glucose *is* abnormally low, there must be a reason for it. The ideal treatment depends on discovering that reason.

SUMMARY

Let's review the points we have covered thus far:

1. Hypoglycemia means a level of blood glucose too low for normal function.
2. Brain function is especially dependent on adequate levels of glucose in the blood.
3. The symptoms of hypoglycemia are not specific; other problems can produce the same feelings and malfunctions.
4. Many people who have been told by well-meaning physicians that they have hypoglycemia may in fact not be suffering from that condition at all.
5. Hypoglycemia is not a disease; it is a manifestation of a disease, toward which diagnosis and treatment should be directed.

Our next chapter will discuss the symptoms which hypoglycemia can cause, since symptoms are usually what prompts patients to seek out a physician in the first place.

2

What Are the Symptoms of Hypoglycemia?

Symptoms are feelings and experiences, such as pain or headache or cramps or nausea. They are what the patient "goes through," and then explains to the doctor. The types of symptoms caused by low blood sugar fall into two broad categories: neuroglycopenic and adrenergic. Don't be scared off by those words.

Neuroglycopenia is the medical term for lack of glucose in the nervous system. *Neuro* refers to the nervous system (brain, spinal cord, and nerves); *glyco* means "glucose"; and *penia* signifies "shortage." Neuroglycopenia is thus a critical lack of glucose in the nervous system. This causes malfunction of the nervous system, and certain feelings and experiences, all of which are called *neuroglycopenic* symptoms.

The other main symptoms caused by hypoglycemia result not from the lack of glucose itself but from the attempts of the body to bring the blood sugar back up to normal. In order to combat hypoglycemia and restore the blood glucose to normal levels, various glands within the body secrete substances into the bloodstream that raise blood glucose. These substances, or hormones, include adrenalin as well as cortisol, glucagon, and growth hormone. Adrenalin (also known as epinephrine) causes racing of the heartbeat, sweating, dilation of the pupils, feelings of alarm and apprehension, and shakiness. The shakiness is sometimes detected as a rapid tremor of the hands or a quiver in the voice or in the knees, but is often just an internal sensation of quivering or "feeling shaky." Because *adrenalin* is involved in the production of these symptoms, they are called *adrenergic* symptoms.

Thus, the two main types of symptoms caused by an abnormally low blood sugar are termed *neuroglycopenic* and *adrenergic*. The neuroglycopenic symptoms result from lack of sufficient glucose and the adrenergic symptoms are by-products of the body's attempts to correct that deficiency.

When their blood sugar is low, some people experience mostly neuroglycopenic symptoms; others have mostly adrenergic symptoms. Depending on how low the blood sugar goes, still other people experience both types of symptoms. The following examples will help you appreciate what it can be like to have the blood sugar level fall below normal.

As a medical intern I was working late one Friday night in a hospital emergency room when Mrs. Sullivan, an elderly woman, came in from a nursing home. The report that accompanied her stated that about two hours earlier she had lost her ability to speak and to use her right arm and leg. The nurses at the nursing home had concluded that Mrs. Sullivan was having a stroke, which is a malfunction of the brain caused by blockage of an artery supplying the brain with blood and oxygen. The symptoms described in their report certainly sounded like a stroke, but when I examined her, Mrs. Sullivan spoke perfectly well and had the use of both of her arms and both of her legs. My examination of her nervous system showed no abnormality.

One can begin to feel a bit paranoid in a busy emergency room at 11:30 P.M. on a Friday night, and the thought crossed my tired mind that perhaps the personnel at the nursing home were just trying to get rid of a patient for the weekend by shipping her into the hospital. I'm afraid a note of annoyance may have crept into my voice as I called the staff at the nursing home, explained that Mrs. Sullivan's nervous system was working perfectly well, and said that I was sending her back to them.

The next night around 11:30 P.M. Mrs. Sullivan was back in the emergency room. The report from the nursing home again described impaired speech and difficulty in using her right arm. A resident physician saw her in the emergency room and took a careful history. He discovered she had mild diabetes. Diabetes involves abnormally high levels of blood sugar and is often treated with drugs that lower the blood glucose. Mrs. Sullivan was taking one of these drugs, known as chlorpropamide (sold as Diabinese). This is a long-acting medication, which can lower the blood glucose for 36 hours or more. She took a 250-mg pill of chlorpropamide every morning but for the past week had not been eating well. When the resident doctor ordered a test of her blood sugar, he uncovered the cause of her problem: hypoglycemia. He therefore gave her an intravenous injection of glucose, and her garbled speech and weak right arm returned promptly to normal.

Her nervous system, now receiving its essential supply of glucose, was functioning normally again. The symptoms of weakness and slurred speech were due to hypoglycemia, and were neuroglycopenic in nature. The blood sugar had fallen because food intake, which raises blood glucose levels, had declined to the point that it no longer balanced the glucose-lowering effect of the chlorpropamide.

The portions of her brain that controlled speech and the movements of her right arm and leg were the first to malfunction when her blood glucose levels dropped. Presumably, since those areas are close together in the brain and supplied by the same artery, there was marginal blood flow to that region of her brain. When the supply of glucose to that portion of the brain became insufficient to support normal function, she lost her speech and the movement of her right limbs. These neuroglycopenic symptoms disappeared as soon as the blood sugar level was raised to normal.

If Mrs. Sullivan's blood sugar had fallen further, additional symptoms would eventually have appeared. Neuroglycopenia can manifest itself as virtually any malfunction of the nervous system, ranging from impaired movement, speech, thought, judgment, sensation, or consciousness, to behavioral and psychological disturbances.

I first met Steve when he was having a seizure, or convulsion, in the psychiatric ward of a large hospital. This 11-year-old boy was on the floor writhing and shaking uncontrollably, with his eyes rolled back and his head turned to the side. I had to sit on him in order to steady his arm enough to get a needle into his vein. Through the needle I drew some blood and gave him an injection of concentrated sugar dissolved in water. He immediately relaxed, stopped shaking, and regained consciousness within the next minute.

Steve had been unaware of what was happening. His roommate said he was usually pleasant but had been belligerent and disagreeable about half an hour earlier and had started swearing and yelling just before he went into the seizure. The nurses working in the psychiatric unit reported that he was usually very cooperative, but occasionally became cranky and uncooperative and foul-mouthed. One nurse had noticed that if she fed him a snack he became calmer again and easier to manage.

Further inquiry disclosed that Steve had been living in a foster home, and his parents reported that he was usually very polite and cooperative, but had occasional, severe, unexpected outbursts of bad temper, foul language, and destructive behavior. It was this behavior that had led to his admission to the psychiatric unit.

What made Steve's story intriguing was that he was a diabetic, taking two injections of insulin a day. Insulin lowers the blood sugar. Too low a blood sugar, because of too much insulin, had caused malfunction of his nervous system, resulting in convulsions.

The blood I had drawn from his vein just before injecting the glucose solution was sent to the laboratory for measurement of blood sugar. The level was 18—definitely hypoglycemic.

We decided to reduce his dosage of insulin and to measure his blood sugar whenever he started having behavioral problems. We found that his behavioral problems were often associated with low blood glucose levels and that further reduction in his doses of insulin virtually eliminated them. Moreover, a glass of orange juice, or some other snack of quickly absorbable carbohydrate, such as a candy bar, could promptly put an end to one of his bad moods. This result of eating sugar is to be expected when symptoms are due to hypoglycemia.

Although most behavior problems are not related to hypoglycemia, in this instance low blood sugar caused some of his symptoms. As you would expect, supplying sugar promptly relieved the problem by raising the blood sugar back to normal.

Not all of the neuroglycopenic manifestations of hypoglycemia are reversible. If the blood glucose is low enough for a long time, permanent brain damage, or even death, can result. The following example of an unfortunate drug addict illustrates this fact.

The emergency-room physician of a large urban hospital called my office to ask if I would assume responsibility for the care of a patient with severe hypoglycemia. He was in a coma when brought to the emergency room, and in accord with standard practice, blood was taken for glucose measurement and intravenous glucose was given. He did not wake up, even though his blood glucose level rose.

The patient was a habitual abuser of drugs. His wife said he would purchase whatever pills he could on the street and take them indiscriminately. The day before, he had purchased a bottle full of blue pills. The vendor had claimed they were "blue codeines." Blood tests later showed the drug to be chlorpropamide, the same drug Mrs. Sullivan and other diabetics use to lower blood sugar.

He had swallowed the entire bottle of pills around noon on Wednesday, and by bedtime that night he was stuporous. Since this was not an unusual condition for him, his wife was not alarmed. The next morning, however, she couldn't rouse him, and when she tried again after lunchtime, he was still out cold. She then became concerned and had him brought by ambulance to the emergency room, where his hypoglycemia was discovered.

By treating this man intensively with intravenous glucose, and later with feedings through a tube into his stomach, we were able to keep his blood sugar consistently normal or above normal. He did regain a measure of consciousness, but remained an apparent "vegetable," unable to speak, walk, or feed himself. Although he didn't die from his prolonged episode of very low blood sugar, he never fully recovered from it. Hours of severe hypoglycemia from his massive overdose of chlorpropamide had permanently damaged his nervous system.

At this point it is important to reiterate that the neuroglycopenic symptoms of hypoglycemia are *not specific.* They are not unique to hypoglycemia. Low blood glucose is not the only cause of malfunction of the nervous system. Most elderly people who suddenly lose their ability to speak and to use their right arm and leg are indeed having a stroke and not suffering from hypoglycemia. Most child behavior problems have no relation to blood sugar levels. Most cases of coma and most seizures are not hypoglycemic in origin. Each of these problems can be caused by hypoglycemia, however, and this possibility should always be considered by the physician while assessing a patient with malfunction of the nervous system.

I thought I was dealing with a case of hypoglycemia once when I took care of a 23-year-old drug addict in the emergency room. His skin was deep yellow from a severe case of hepatitis, and his face was twitching and contorted. He was fully conscious. His back and neck muscles were in spasm, so he had a peculiar arched posture.

By this time I was a resident physician and was aware that very severe hepatitis can cause hypoglycemia. Hepatitis is a state of liver damage and is sometimes called yellow jaundice because of a yellow pigment, normally excreted by the liver, that accumulates in the skin and eyeballs of the patient. I was aware that the liver is necessary for the maintenance of normal blood glucose levels, and that in severe liver damage the blood glucose level may fall abnormally low and cause neuroglycopenic symptoms, perhaps like those I was observing.

I quickly inserted a needle into this patient's vein and drew a blood sample for glucose measurement, then gave him generous amounts of intravenous glucose solution. To my disappointment, his muscle contortions continued. Later the pretreatment blood glucose report came back as 84—perfectly normal. No wonder his condition hadn't improved from the intravenous glucose. But why was his nervous system malfunctioning? As he recounted his recent history, I learned the answer.

Three days earlier he had come to the emergency room complaining of nausea, a frequent symptom of hepatitis. To control his nausea he had been given a prescription of a drug named perphenazine, to be taken by rectal suppository. He had taken quite a few of these suppositories the day I met him in his contorted condition, and he was suffering one of the known side effects of perphenazine. Fortunately for him, an antidote was readily available. I gave him a slow intravenous injection of diphenhydramine, a drug that counteracts that particular side effect of perphenazine, and his symptoms immediately vanished. This case illustrates several basic and important points.

His symptoms could conceivably have been caused by hypoglycemia, but in fact they were not. The diagnosis of hypoglycemia could not be reliably made just on the basis of the symptoms alone, since they are not specific for that condition. One must measure the blood sugar and find it abnormally low before concluding that the patient's symptoms may be due to hypoglycemia.

The proper treatment of this patient's symptoms depended upon first arriving at the correct diagnosis. Intravenous glucose and dietary modification don't help correct this reaction to perphenazine nearly as well as an injection of diphenhydramine does. Intelligent diagnosis precedes intelligent treatment.

Since the neuroglycopenic symptoms of hypoglycemia are *not specific* for low blood glucose, the symptoms alone are not sufficient to make an intelligent diagnosis. This same fact applies also to the adrenergic symptoms of hypoglycemia.

If you were walking alone down a dark alley at night and suddenly someone jumped out at you from the shadows, brandishing a knife and screaming, you would undoubtedly experience a surge of adrenalin in your bloodstream. Adrenalin, or epinephrine, is a hormone secreted from the adrenal glands into the bloodstream in response to a variety of stresses. These stresses include sudden fright, hypoglycemia, massive bleeding, and several other conditions. Adrenalin makes the heart pound forcefully and rapidly. The skin gets clammy and the hands may tremble. You may feel a quiver in your knees, or you may just feel "shaky" inside. For example, think back to when you had to give a speech in public —a stress that causes many people to experience adrenergic symptoms. You may have had some of these feelings. These symptoms are caused by substances (mainly epinephrine) secreted into your bloodstream during stress. Because epinephrine, or *adrenalin,* causes these feelings, we call them *adrenergic* symptoms.

The outpouring of adrenalin responsible for these alarming symptoms can be caused by hypoglycemia. But they can also be triggered by a variety of other stresses and conditions. Too many people make the mistake of concluding they must have hypoglycemia because they have these adrenergic symptoms.

Just as the smoke and flames of a forest fire don't tell you whether it was started by a cigarette, a campfire, or a bolt of lightning, adrenergic symptoms themselves don't tell you what triggered the sudden outpouring of adrenalin. Once a forest fire is burning, it can look and smell and feel the same, no matter what started the combustion in the first place. The following case history illustrates the point that adrenergic symptoms are *not specific* for hypoglycemia.

A Chinese man in his 30s experienced frequent episodes of pounding heartbeat, sweating, and headache. During these spells a feeling of dread would come over him. He said, "I feel as though I am going to die." Because his symptoms sounded adrenergic, we measured his adrenalin levels during an attack and found them to be very high. That led us to the next question: *Why* were this man's adrenal glands secreting so much epinephrine? Perhaps the cause was hypoglycemia.

We measured his blood glucose levels during several of these attacks, but they ranged always on the high side of normal. He did not have hypoglycemia.

What he did have was a tumor on his left adrenal gland. This tumor was making and secreting large amounts of epinephrine, which in turn was giving him high blood sugar, high blood pressure, headache, sweating, and rapid heartbeat.

An operation was done to remove the tumor from his left adrenal gland. After the operation his adrenergic symptoms disappeared, and his blood sugar and blood pressure promptly returned to normal. His symptoms had indeed been due to adrenalin, but hypoglycemia was not involved at all.

Hypoglycemia is often experienced by diabetic patients taking medications such as insulin or chlorpropamide to lower the blood glucose. These patients report the entire gamut of neurologic and adrenergic symptoms. Among my diabetic patients taking insulin, the most frequently reported symptom of hypoglycemia is a "shaky" feeling inside, often accompanied by perspiration. Patients learn to recognize these early adrenergic symptoms of hypoglycemia, and to prevent them from worsening by eating some carbohydrate to bring the blood sugar level quickly back to normal. They may then reduce their dosage of insulin, and never experience the more severe symptoms of hypoglycemia. Three commonly occurring situations, however, may prevent diabetic patients from experiencing the adrenergic warning symptoms of low blood sugar, so that a neuroglycopenic problem such as confusion or incoordination may be the first symptoms they experience as their blood glucose falls too low. These three situations are:

1. very gradual lowering of the blood glucose level, seen especially with the use of long-acting types of insulin,
2. usage of drugs that block the action of adrenalin, and
3. severe nerve damage from long-standing diabetes.

An explanation of each of these three problems follows:

Gradual descent of blood glucose levels. Steve, the 11-year-old boy described earlier in this chapter, whom I met while he was having a seizure, was taking only the long-acting forms of insulin. These are absorbed slowly and lower the blood sugar more gradually than the quick-acting types of insulin. In some patients they cause little in the way of adrenergic symptoms.

The rate of fall of the blood glucose, in addition to the actual level of blood glucose itself, appears to be a factor in initiating the outpouring of adrenalin and other hormones antagonistic to the hypoglycemic action of insulin. Thus, most people experience adrenergic symptoms when blood glucose levels fall below normal if the rate of fall of blood glucose is quite rapid. When the descent of blood glucose levels is very gradual, however, they may experience few or no adrenergic symptoms at all. Their first symptoms may be change in personality or behavior, incoordination, double or blurred vision, or some other neuroglycopenic manifestation. This may also be the case even in instances of hypoglycemia not caused by treatment for diabetes. For example, the case of a man with an insulin-secreting tumor of the pancreas will be described in Chapter 7. He showed this pattern of neuroglycopenic but no adrenergic symptoms apparently because of a very gradual decline in his blood glucose levels.

Drugs that block adrenalin. The actions of adrenalin on body tissues may be blocked by certain drugs, such as propranolol and metoprolol. These drugs may prevent the patient from experiencing the tremor and rapid heartbeat that adrenalin, secreted in response to low blood glucose levels, would otherwise elicit. I saw a dramatic example of this during my residency training.

A diabetic patient in his 40s, unconscious and convulsing, arrived by ambulance in the emergency room of our hospital. A Medic-Alert bracelet on his wrist identified him as a diabetic who was taking insulin. It took five doctors and nurses to restrain him enough to insert an intravenous catheter so we could draw blood for glucose measurement and give him intravenous glucose. He stopped convulsing and promptly regained consciousness after we gave him 25 grams of glucose by vein. He then recalled that he had felt weak at work that morning and a little hungry about 11:00 A.M. He said he had felt "not quite right" and the last thing he remembered was reaching into his coat pocket for one of the sugar cubes he kept there for correction of low blood sugar. The sugar cubes were still in his pocket when he arrived at the emergency room. He had evidently passed out before he got to them. Then the reason for his lack of warning symptoms became clear.

He related that he was taking rather large doses of the drug propranolol for his high blood pressure. He had taken his propranolol that morning as usual, as well as his insulin. Since propranolol prevents the tremor and speeding of the heartbeat caused by adrenalin, he hadn't had those warning symptoms to help him realize he should raise his blood glucose level by eating a sugar lump. By the time he recognized any symptoms at all, he was about to lose consciousness because of neuroglycopenia.

Drugs like metoprolol probably do not cause hypoglycemia, but they do mask its adrenergic symptoms. They should therefore be used with caution in diabetic patients taking medication that lowers the blood sugar.

These adrenalin-blocking drugs, sometimes called "beta-blockers," are becoming very widely used in the treatment of conditions such as migraine headache, hyperthyroidism, high blood pressure, glaucoma, and irregularity of the heartbeat. Moreover, because they do prevent adrenergic symptoms, they are sometimes quite useful in preventing or relieving adrenergic symptoms that are due to causes other than hypoglycemia.

Diabetic nerve damage. In cases of diabetes mellitus of long duration, many of the nerves in the body become damaged. Once damaged, they may no longer carry the electrical impulses that register pain or other sensations. Among the nerves that may be damaged in diabetes are those that control the functions of internal organs, such as the motions of the intestines, the slowing and speeding of the heartbeat, the contraction of blood vessels, and the release of adrenalin from the adrenal glands. Consequently, people who have had diabetes for many years may experience intestinal problems or a drop in blood pressure when they stand up. They may also lack the normal adrenalin response to low blood sugar. They are, of course, still liable to have the neuroglycopenic manifestations of hypoglycemia, even though they may lack the adrenalin secretion necessary to produce the adrenergic symptoms.

Before closing this chapter I want to add a final detail to the categories of symptoms caused by hypoglycemia. In addition to neuroglycopenic and adrenergic symptoms, in rare instances low blood sugar causes a third type of experience, known as angina pectoris. "Angina," as it is called for short, is a pain in the chest, often described as a heavy pressure discomfort. Sometimes it is felt in the neck or shoulders or arms. Its usual cause is lack of sufficient oxygen supply to the heart, because of a blockage or spasm of the coronary arteries, which supply blood to the heart. Patients with blockage of these arteries are likely to experience angina during exercise, which increases the need for oxygen in the heart. Such people may also feel angina during hypoglycemia. It is not known whether the angina is caused directly by a lack of glucose to supply the energy needs of the heart or indirectly through adrenalin causing the heart to beat faster and thus use more oxygen. In any event, angina pectoris, though usually unrelated to the level of blood sugar, can be triggered by hypoglycemia.

SUMMARY

To summarize the main points of this chapter:

1. Hypoglycemia causes neuroglycopenic symptoms due to malfunction of the nervous system.
2. Hypoglycemia causes adrenergic symptoms due to the release of adrenalin as the body attempts to restore the blood sugar to normal.
3. Rarely, hypoglycemia causes chest pain in persons with blockage of the coronary arteries.
4. None of these symptoms are specific for hypoglycemia. They can be caused by many other conditions besides low blood sugar.
5. In certain instances, such as when adrenalin-blocking drugs are being used, the adrenergic symptoms of hypoglycemia may not be experienced, and neuroglycopenic symptoms may be the first to appear.

Now that the reader is familiar with some of the symptoms that hypoglycemia may cause, the next question is this: How low does your blood sugar have to go before it causes you to have symptoms and your nervous system to malfunction?

3

How Low Is Too Low?

When we speak of a "level" of blood sugar, we are really talking about concentration—how much sugar is dissolved in a certain volume of blood. When the blood sugar level is low, there is not much sugar dissolved in the blood.

You will notice that the units of blood glucose measurement are metric. The amount of glucose is given in milligrams and the amount of blood in deciliters. Milligrams per deciliter is abbreviated mg/dl. When you think that a milligram is one one-thousandth of a gram, and there are 5 grams in a U.S. nickel, and that a deciliter is just a little more than 3 fluid ounces, you realized that we are talking about minuscule amounts of this essential fuel. Even at normal levels of blood glucose, the sugar is not concentrated enough to taste sweet, as you know if you have ever cut your lip or your tongue.

There is a widespread misconception that levels of blood glucose below 70 mg/dl are abnormally low. This misunderstanding has probably arisen from the fact that most laboratory report sheets list a so-called normal range for plasma glucose of around 70–110 mg/dl or 70–120 mg/dl. What is so often overlooked is that this is the normal range for blood glucose after a 12-to-14-hour fast, and is defined in such a way as to include only 95% of normal values.

After you eat, your blood sugar normally rises somewhat as sugar is absorbed from your intestine into the bloodstream. Your blood sugar then comes down, and in many people drops below 70 mg/dl with no ill-effects whatever. This drop below 70 mg/dl is especially likely to occur when a very sugary meal is taken, such as during an oral glucose tolerance test. The pitfalls of oral glucose tolerance testing have been the source of much of the misunderstanding about hypoglycemia, and are explained in Chapter 5.

Under normal day-to-day circumstances, people need a blood sugar level of at least 35–40 mg/dl to function normally. A blood glucose concentration below that level will cause most people to experience some symptoms or abnormality of body function.

Careful studies of the level of blood glucose at which symptoms appear have been carried out in patients with diseases causing hypoglycemia, and also in normal persons made hypoglycemic experimentally. Both types of studies reach the same conclusion: Symptoms start appearing as the blood glucose level falls below 40 mg/dl.[1–3]

Between the levels of 40 and 55 mg/dl, some people will experience symptoms, but others will not. This may therefore be regarded as a "gray zone" in which the blood sugar level may or may not be responsible for the symptoms a patient is experiencing.

Levels of blood sugar down to but above 55 mg/dl are so commonly found in normal people without any symptoms at all of hypoglycemia that it is unlikely that they are ever truly responsible for symptoms in anyone.

The limits of the normal, "gray-zone," and abnormal ranges for blood sugar depend on the laboratory methods being used to make the measurement. If the red blood cells are separated from the rest of the blood before the measurement of sugar is made, the reading is called a "plasma" or "serum" glucose level. Since the red cells do not contain quite as much glucose as the plasma, a plasma glucose reading comes out about 10–15% higher than a whole blood glucose measurement. Modern automated laboratory equipment usually measures glucose in plasma or serum. In such instances, the cutoff between definitely low and "gray-zone" levels shifts upward to 40–45 mg/dl, and the upper limit of the "gray zone" reaches to about 60 mg/dl.

Under certain special circumstances the body can function normally with an even lower blood glucose than those outlined above for ordinary day-to-day living. These exceptional circumstances include:

[1] **F. J. Service et al., *Mayo Clinic Proceedings* 51 (1976), 417.**
[2] **V. Marks, *British Medical Journal* 1 (1972), 430.**
[3] **D. D. Johnson et al., *Journal of the American Medical Association* 243, 1151.**

1. being a newborn baby;
2. fasting for several days, especially in women and children;
3. exercising strenuously for a long time, such as running a marathon.

During the first 72 hours of life, newborn babies appear to function normally with blood sugar levels below the adult range. This has caused some controversy as to what levels should be regarded as hypoglycemic at this tender age. Most authorities believe that levels down to 30 mg/dl can be normal in the first 72 hours of life in a normal-sized, full-term infant, and that levels in the 20s may be normal in a premature baby. There is no firm proof that levels this low are harmless, however, even though they occur frequently. Since babies don't explain their symptoms to their doctors in a very detailed manner, arguments about how low is too low in infancy will doubtless continue. In any event, no lasting harm appears to result from these levels.

When healthy adult men fast for 72 hours, their blood glucose levels often fall into the low 50s with no evidence of malfunction or symptoms. Interestingly enough, their levels do not drop below 50 mg/dl.[4,5] In healthy adult women, on the other hand, blood glucose levels have been shown to fall as low as the 20s with no evidence of hypoglycemia (i.e., no symptoms and no brain malfunction).[4] It isn't that the women can't make more sugar while fasting, since they do raise their blood glucose when exercised at the end of the 72-hour fast.[5] Women simply appear to be better than men at switching over to a reliance on fat, instead of sugar, as a fuel during fasting.[4]

An important scientific study recently conducted at Yale University Medical School showed that levels of plasma glucose as low as 25 mg/dl to 45 mg/dl are frequently found during extreme and prolonged physical exertion, without causing any symptoms or impairment of function.[6] The research team wanted to clarify whether the phenomenon known as "hitting the wall"—a severe tiredness that affects many marathon runners about 20 miles into the race—was due to hypoglycemia. Their results show conclusively that glucose levels as low as 25–45 mg/dl can be achieved during exercise, but that preventing the glucose levels from falling

[4] **T. J. Merimee and J. E. Tyson, *New England Journal of Medicine* 291 (1974), 1275.**
[5] **S. S. Fajans and J. C. Floyd, *New England Journal of Medicine* 294 (1976), 766.**
[6] **P. Felig et al., *New England Journal of Medicine* 306 (1982), 895.**

(by intake of carbohydrate) had no effect whatsoever on symptoms or performance. These scientists have thus shown that the range of normal blood glucose is somewhat lower during the extreme stress of prolonged exercise, as it may be also during the stress of a newborn baby leaving its mother's womb, and during prolonged fasting in a woman. Presumably, the body depends on other fuels, such as ketones, during such times.

One other stressful circumstance causes low levels of blood glucose in healthy persons: the glucose tolerance test. As will be discussed in detail in Chapter 5, blood glucose levels often fall below 50 mg/dl during this very artificial procedure. Some observers have noted that symptoms occur in most subjects with blood glucose levels under 45 mg/dl during the test,[7] while others have disputed this claim.[3] Detailed studies show, however, that symptoms correlate very poorly with blood glucose levels during the stressful setting of a glucose tolerance test.[8]

Some people have no symptoms at all at a level of blood glucose that would produce symptoms in others. This fact accounts for the "gray zone" of glucose levels, in which some people are hypoglycemic while others, with an identical concentration of blood sugar, are not. While one person may be perfectly unaffected by a blood glucose of 42 mg/dl, another could have definite symptoms at the same level. Even within the same person, one part of the brain may function perfectly well at a level of blood sugar that is too low for other parts of the brain. For example, the gray matter on the surface, which is involved in reasoning and speech and fine muscle control, needs more glucose than portions of the interior that control the rate of breathing. The drug addict mentioned in Chapter 2, for example, continued to breathe normally even while unconscious.

Regional differences in blood supply may also cause certain parts of the brain to require a higher concentration of glucose than is needed for other areas of the brain. For example, if a person has hardening and narrowing of the artery supplying blood to a certain portion of the brain—such as the speech center or the vision center—a lowering of the blood glucose to a level of 55 mg/dl

[7] **M. A. Permutt, J. Delmez, and W. Stenson, *Journal of Clinical Endocrinology and Metabolism* 43 (1976), 1088.**

[8] **V. Marks, "Hypoglycemia: Proceedings of the European Symposium Rome," *Hormone and Metabolic Research* (Suppl. 6) (Stuttgart: Georg Thieme Publishers, 1976), 1.**

may result in glucose deficiency for that part of the brain. The result would be hypoglycemic symptoms such as garbled speech or blurred vision, reflecting the malfunction of the part of the brain with a borderline supply of blood. This was probably the case with Mrs. Sullivan, whose story is recounted early in Chapter 2.

Remember that the rate of delivery of glucose to a tissue depends *both* on the rate of blood flow to that tissue *and* on the concentration of glucose in the blood. It's just like the supply of oxygen to a deep-sea diver; his getting enough oxygen depends on both the rate of flow and the concentration of oxygen in his air line.

Thus, there is no single specific concentration of blood glucose that in all circumstances cleanly divides levels that are always high enough from those that are definitely too low.

As an endocrinologist, I sometimes *intentionally* make certain patients hypoglycemic as part of a diagnostic test called an *insulin tolerance test* (not to be confused with glucose tolerance test). The purpose of the test is to see whether the patient's pituitary gland is healthy, since a healthy pituitary gland will secrete certain hormones under the stress of hypoglycemia. The test includes an intravenous injection of insulin, which causes the blood glucose level to fall. We purposely give enough insulin to make the blood glucose go lower than normal. Then we see whether the pituitary can respond by secreting its hormones. In order for the test to be valid, we have to get the blood sugar down to definitely low levels. For this reason we insist on getting the plasma glucose down to 40 mg/dl or less (i.e., under 36 mg/dl if blood rather than plasma glucose is being measured). If only enough insulin is given to get the plasma glucose down to, say, 50 mg/dl, we cannot be certain we have truly produced hypoglycemia, and therefore cannot be sure we have stimulated the pituitary gland sufficiently to have a valid test of its ability to secrete its hormones.[9] Some people do respond to plasma glucose levels in the gray area above 40 mg/dl, but we cannot be sure, on the basis of the glucose measurement alone, of having achieved hypoglycemia unless the plasma glucose falls below 40 mg/dl.

Likewise, in everyday life, plasma glucose levels between 40 and 60 mg/dl may be abnormally low in some cases, but to be certain of hypoglycemia on the basis of the glucose level alone,

[9] **G. M. Besser and C. R. W. Edwards, *Clinic in Endocrinology and Metabolism* 1, no. 2 (1972), 466.**

you must have a plasma level under 40 mg/dl. Even then you must exclude the exceptional circumstances reviewed earlier in this chapter (the newborn state, glucose tolerance tests, prolonged exercise, prolonged fasting in women) before settling on a diagnosis of hypoglycemia based solely on a blood glucose level under 40 mg/dl. In the "gray zone" above 40 mg/dl, you must be even more cautious about deciding on a diagnosis of hypoglycemia. To conclude that a level of 50 mg/dl is hypoglycemic for a given individual requires repeated observation of hypoglycemic symptoms whenever the blood glucose falls that low, and the absence of those symptoms when the glucose level is higher.

The following example illustrates how the significance of blood glucose levels in the "gray zone" was clarified in the case of an actual patient, whom we shall call Kara.

Kara had diabetes mellitus, a disease in which the blood glucose level is abnormally high. Twice each day Kara gave herself injections of insulin, which lowers the blood sugar level. It was the lack of insulin in Kara's body that caused her blood glucose levels to be higher than normal. By injecting herself with insulin, Kara could bring her blood glucose level back down toward normal.

Unfortunately, like many people who take insulin for diabetes, Kara sometimes took too much. This caused episodes of low blood sugar. Shortly after beginning insulin treatment at the age of 23, Kara experienced severe hypoglycemia, with symptoms of rapid heartbeat, sweating, shakiness, then mental confusion and loss of consciousness. This experience so frightened her that she became "gun-shy" regarding the use of insulin.

To avoid such symptoms of hypoglycemia, Kara began to use doses of insulin that were too small to bring her glucose level down to normal. This resulted in her having continued symptoms of poorly controlled diabetes, including weight loss, excessive thirst, and profuse urination. She lost 40 pounds and became severely underweight and very weak. It was essential to her health that she take more insulin, to correct her continuing downhill slide. Her physician therefore told her to take larger doses of insulin.

Each time Kara would take an increased dose of insulin, however, she was anxious and would notice rapid heartbeat and some sweating. This made her feel sure she was beginning another episode of hypoglycemia. Since anxiety (in this case from concern about hypoglycemia) can cause these adrenergic symptoms, it became very confusing to Kara and her physician as to whether she was really having spells of low blood glucose or just having spells of anxiety because she was so afraid of low blood glucose.

This problem was finally solved by putting Kara in the hospital, and increasing her insulin dosage. Whenever Kara became anxious or sweaty or felt her heart starting to race, the laboratory technician was immediately called to draw blood for glucose measurement. It soon became evident that most of Kara's symptoms were occurring at blood glucose levels far *above* normal and were therefore not due to hypoglycemia at all. With this reassurance that her blood glucose was not even close to levels that could produce unconsciousness or other serious problems, Kara calmed down. The anxiety attacks stopped. She became able to take insulin in doses adequate to bring her blood sugar toward normal. This allowed her weight loss to cease and her thirst and excessive urination to abate. She started to feel much better.

A few mornings later she went for a long walk around the hospital. She had skipped her breakfast that morning because she just couldn't face the day's hospital fare of oatmeal mush, cold eggs, and dry wheat toast. She had taken her usual insulin dose, and this, combined with decreased food intake and increased exercise, all teamed up to lower her blood glucose into the hypoglycemic range. She started to feel weak, shaky, and sweaty and to have blurred vision. She realized this wasn't just one of her old anxiety attacks, so she called for the nurse. The nurse called the lab technician to come immediately to draw blood for glucose measurement, and then gave her a big glass of orange juice with two teaspoons of sugar stirred in. This relieved her symptoms within a few minutes. Then the report came back from the laboratory—the blood glucose had been 52 mg/dl. Two similar episodes occurred in the next two days, each time with relief of symptoms following orange juice, and with blood sugars measured at 41 and 46 mg/dl, again in the "gray zone." These symptoms were probably due to hypoglycemia. Not only were the symptoms typical of hypoglycemia, but they were relieved by sugar intake, and the blood sugar levels were low enough to possibly cause the symptoms. It is this correlation of symptoms, blood glucose measurements, and the effects of glucose administration that allows us to sort out the significance of blood sugar levels in the "gray zone."

Kara learned to recognize her symptoms of hypoglycemia, and

they became a valuable guide in helping her adjust her insulin dosage correctly. She had overcome her anxiety and was able to recognize symptoms of hypoglycemia, thanks to the measurements of her blood sugar during the symptoms in question.

Kara's case makes it easy to see the importance of *accurate* and *reliable* measurements of the glucose level in plasma or blood. Equipment that, properly used, can measure blood glucose accurately with a less than 5% error is widely available. This equipment, unfortunately, is quite expensive. There is also expense involved in maintaining quality control within a laboratory. It includes running of duplicate specimens to be sure they agree, and testing the equipment with standard solutions and unknown samples. The health departments of some states, for example, periodically mail unknown samples to licensed laboratories within their jurisdiction. The clinical laboratory has to measure the glucose level in the "unknown" and send in its reading by mail to the state reference laboratory. If the clinical laboratory is not getting an accurate reading, its procedures must be corrected until it can consistently come up with the right answers.

One of the most common mistakes in blood glucose measurement involves the improper handling of the blood specimen prior to laboratory analysis. Since the blood cells themselves consume glucose, the blood glucose level in a tube of untreated whole blood will gradually decline. Within a few hours, readings that are falsely low by 20% or 30% may be obtained. I recently saw a patient whose "hypoglycemia" was due to this very problem: Blood had been drawn in a doctor's office and left untreated for hours while being transported to a city miles away, where the laboratory found an abnormally low blood glucose level. Using proper procedures, we proved her blood glucose levels to be consistently normal.

Any of four steps can prevent the problem described in the previous paragraph. First, one can centrifuge the blood so that the cells quickly settle to the bottom of the tube, then separate the plasma from the cells, and store the plasma until the measurement is made. Second, one can draw the blood into a tube containing sodium fluoride, which poisons the cells so they don't consume glucose. Third, freezing the blood or plasma will significantly and satisfactorily slow the process of glucose degradation by cells. Fourth, the laboratory measurement can be run promptly, on freshly drawn blood, before the cells have time to alter the glucose level.

Unfortunately, some doctor's offices use equipment and procedures for blood glucose measurement that are accurate only within about 15%. This includes devices that can be used at home for measurement of blood glucose levels by the patient. Although sufficiently accurate to help greatly in the treatment of diabetes, these devices do not have the degree of accuracy needed to sort out a difficult diagnostic problem with blood sugar levels in or near the "gray zone."

Before leaving this somewhat technical chapter on laboratory measurement, a word of warning is in order: Remember that chemistry laboratories are staffed by human beings. Laboratory tests are therefore not infallible. Although the measurement of blood and plasma glucose levels is relatively straightforward, errors do occur. Before hastily concluding that someone does or does not have hypoglycemia, one must consider the entire picture of symptoms, physical examination, and laboratory tests, sometimes repeating some of the tests and observations. The next chapter gives several more examples of how this was done in actual individual case histories.

SUMMARY

1. Blood glucose levels in adults below 40 mg/dl are generally not normal, and levels greater than 55 mg/dl are not abnormal.
2. When the measurements are made on plasma instead of blood, these boundaries shift upward to about 45 mg/dl and 60 mg/dl.
3. In between, a "gray zone" exists, and diagnosis may depend on correlating symptoms with blood glucose levels, and on the relief of symptoms by raising the blood sugar.
4. The limits of normal for glucose levels are lower in certain exceptional circumstances, including:
   a) the newborn period,
   b) prolonged fasting, especially in women,
   c) severe, prolonged exercise, and
   d) glucose tolerance tests.
5. In measuring blood glucose levels, proper equipment and techniques must be used or results may be inaccurate and misleading.

4

How to Find Out Whether You Have Hypoglycemia

Now let's return to the case of Ernest, the young man we met in the Introduction. The reader should understand by now that the question of whether or not Ernest has hypoglycemia depends on the level of his blood sugar. To figure out whether low blood sugar was causing Ernest's symptoms, we obviously had to measure his blood sugar during the symptoms. The question we had to answer was simply this: When Ernest was having his symptoms, was the blood sugar low enough to explain the symptoms?

To answer this question, I gave Ernest a slip of paper introducing him to the laboratory in the neighborhood where he lived and worked. The slip read: "Please draw blood for glucose measurement whenever the patient comes in and requests it. Note date and time carefully for each specimen."

Since that lab was open only between 7:30 A.M. and 6 P.M., I also gave him a similar slip for the local hospital laboratory, which was open for outpatients 24 hours a day.

I instructed Ernest to have his blood sugar measured at the lab *during symptoms suspected of being due to hypoglycemia,* at least six times in the coming weeks. I also instructed him to keep a notebook log of the symptoms he was having at the time his blood glucose was measured. He was to write down the following items each time his blood was taken for glucose measurement: the date, the time, the symptoms.

He was to return with the notebook a few weeks later, when he would read me the date, time, and symptoms, and I would read back to him the corresponding blood glucose values. In this way we could discover which of his symptoms might be attributable to a low level of blood glucose.

At that point, *if and when* we found the blood glucose to be *low*, we would start an investigation of *why* it was low. First, however, we needed to find out whether he had hypoglycemia at all.

I encouraged him to do the things that provoked his symptoms, so we could make the blood measurements that would allow us to find out whether hypoglycemia was indeed the culprit. In his case, eating sweets was one of the surefire ways to trigger his symptoms.

I happened to have a Hershey chocolate bar in the office, so I gave it to him—to his surprise and mild horror—and sent him across the street to the laboratory to have his blood drawn once the symptoms hit him full-force. He would then record the date, time, and symptoms in his notebook, and our investigation was on its way.

Five weeks later he returned with his notebook log, which read something like this:

"Aug. 9, 11:30 A.M. After eating Hershey bar in doctor's office, felt nervous, tired, and a little shaky, but could think clearly. Not light-headed this time. No headache."

I then read him the results of his blood glucose report, dated August 9 at 11:30 A.M.—it was 104 mg/dl. This is a normal level and provided evidence that his symptoms on August 9 at 11:30 A.M. were not hypoglycemic in nature.[1] The next entry in his log read:

"Aug. 13, 9:20 A.M. No breakfast yet this A.M. Headache. Light-headed. Not clear mentally. A little nervous." The plasma glucose was normal, at 74 mg/dl.

"Aug. 13, 10:35 A.M. Had breakfast at Denny's half hour ago. Headache still there. Can't think or concentrate well. Nervous.

[1] As explained in Chapter 3, plasma glucose levels of 60 or more are not hypoglycemic. Levels under 40 are often abnormally low. Between 40 mg/dl and 60 mg/dl a "gray zone" exists.

Worried about eating so much sugar (pancakes, syrup, and milk). Very tired—can't work today." The plasma glucose was 128 mg/dl.

"Aug. 13, 4:00 P.M. Rested most of day. Still tired. Thinking clearly but no energy." The plasma glucose was 76 mg/dl.

"Aug. 19, 11:10 A.M. Ate 2 Hostess Twinkies on my break half hour ago. Now feeling light-headed, nervous, can't concentrate." Plasma glucose 103 mg/dl.

"Aug. 29, 5:42 P.M. Feeling fine. Just thought I'd see what my sugar is when I'm not feeling bad." Plasma glucose 87 mg/dl.

"Aug. 30, 7:38 A.M. No breakfast today. Haven't eaten since 7:00 P.M. last night. Feel OK." Plasma glucose 68 mg/dl.

"Sept. 4, 2:05 P.M. Late lunch today. Very tired. Not working or concentrating well. Slight headache." Plasma glucose 95 mg/dl.

"Sept. 4, 9:55 A.M. Nothing to eat since yesterday noon. Feel dizzy but no headache or nervousness." Plasma glucose 72 mg/dl.

"Sept. 4, 10:27 A.M. Feel sick to my stomach, nervous, dizzy after eating 2 Three Musketeers. Shaky." Plasma glucose 147 mg/dl.

All of these glucose levels were normal—not even in the borderline range. We thus had no evidence of hypoglycemia, and no reason to think that hypoglycemia could explain his symptoms or that treatment for any of the causes of hypoglycemia would be beneficial.

The fact that Ernest had initially felt better while following a "hypoglycemic diet" in no way proves that he had hypoglycemia, since symptoms often come and go spontaneously. Moreover, any treatment, from aspirin to spinal manipulation to acupuncture to surgery to snake oil or sugar pills, may alleviate symptoms through a placebo effect. Mental suggestion can be powerful medicine, but cannot always substitute for intelligent diagnosis and treatment. Thus, the response to his diet was not firm evidence in favor of hypoglycemia. Indeed, while adhering ever more strictly to his diet, his condition had worsened. This realization helped Ernest accept the fact that he did not have hypoglycemia after all.

I made a tentative diagnosis of malnutrition, underweight, and anxiety neurosis. With counseling and reassurance, and with reintroduction of normal food intake, Ernest gradually regained his lost weight and felt better. By discarding the mistaken diagnosis of hypoglycemia, we were able to move on to more helpful measures.

In order to verify or disprove the diagnosis of hypoglycemia, it is useful, and often necessary, to provoke the symptoms in question. This allows us to investigate the symptoms, though it often requires resourceful tactics in order to produce the symptoms at a time and place where blood glucose can be measured.

For example, Melissa's story was of a flushed, giddy feeling experienced only after eating a hot fudge sundae from a certain ice-cream store in Palo Alto, California. Hot fudge sundaes from Farrell's (a popular chain of ice-cream parlors in the western United States), however, did not produce the symptoms. To test the possibility that her symptoms were due to hypoglycemia, as Melissa and her family felt they were, I had her go to the ice-cream store in Palo Alto and order a hot fudge sundae to take out. She was then to drive to a laboratory and eat the sundae sitting in the car in the parking lot. As soon as the symptoms came on, she was to leave her car, go into the lab, and have her blood drawn for glucose measurement. She carried out the experiment as directed, and had a perfectly normal blood glucose of 110 mg/dl while feeling flushed and giddy from her hot fudge sundae.

Patrick O'Grady presented an even more interesting challenge. His single symptom was loss of consciousness. His family physician suspected hypoglycemia and referred him for evaluation of this possibility. Obviously, in order to determine whether his symptoms were due to hypoglycemia, we would have liked to have the opportunity to measure his blood glucose as he was passing out, but this would be virtually impossible to arrange safely. His history, however, opened a means of investigation.

Mr. O'Grady was an excellent athlete, and would often run five to ten miles at a time, or spend two or three hours in an intensive series of racquetball games. Occasionally, while exercising in this manner and having skipped a meal earlier that day, he would pass out with only a few seconds of warning symptoms consisting of faintness and forceful, irregular heartbeat. He admitted that he often felt hungry during his workouts, but would push himself despite this symptom in an attempt to improve his already excellent physical condition. We decided to try to measure his blood sugar before he passed out, reasoning that before he reached a level of blood sugar low enough to produce unconsciousness, he would surely have to get his blood sugar down at least into the borderline range.

We arranged for him to eat only a very light breakfast, skip lunch entirely, then take off work about 2:30 in the afternoon. He changed into his jogging suit and put a candy bar in his pocket to have available in case of severe hunger or faintness. He then followed a five-mile jogging course we had outlined, ending at the laboratory. If at that point he felt no symptoms at all, he was to have his blood glucose drawn, then keep running around the parking lot until his symptoms finally did begin to appear, then get his blood drawn again. The test was carried out as planned, and both blood glucose levels were found to be in the 90s—not even close to the hypoglycemic range.

Another patient, Homer Tennyson, had symptoms of lightheadedness, sweating, palpitations, and blurred vision in the mornings, especially after skipping breakfast. Sometimes it interfered with his driving to work so much that Homer had to pull off the road for fear of having an accident. We thought it would be too dangerous to have him drive to the laboratory in this condition, so he was hospitalized and kept without food for almost 24 hours. When the symptoms appeared, his blood glucose measured 30 mg/dl. This was indeed a case of hypoglycemia. Further investigation of his hypoglycemia showed that Mr. Tennyson had a tumor in his pancreas that was secreting too much insulin—a hormone that lowers the levels of blood sugar. He was cured by an operation to remove the tumor.

In each of these cases, the first question was not *why* the patient had hypoglycemia, but *whether* the patient had hypoglycemia. Therefore, the first step in the evaluation was to *measure the blood glucose during the symptoms*. Then, once the blood glucose was found to be indeed low, specific tests would be needed to determine the particular cause of low blood sugar in this individual. Only after the cause had been determined, could the right treatment be given. Mr. Tennyson, for example, needed an operation on his pancreas to remove an insulin-producing tumor. A new diet wouldn't have helped him. On the other hand, a diet is the correct treatment for certain other causes of hypoglycemia. Until you have an intelligent, specific diagnosis, you are not likely to get intelligent, specific treatment. This principle—diagnosis first, treatment second—is illustrated by the following case.

For thirteen years Sterling Majors carried the diagnosis of hypoglycemia and followed a variety of diets. He was in basically good health, and the diets didn't bother him, but neither did they solve the problem that had sent this 50-year-old athletic business executive to the doctor in the first place. His problem was that he sometimes became very weak and faint on Saturday mornings while playing three to five hours of doubles tennis.

As the symptoms came on, Sterling would suddenly feel so weak he would have to lie down to keep from passing out. On a couple of occasions he actually fainted. His weak, faint feeling was usually accompanied by perspiration, and sometimes by a feeling of rapid heart action. Taking food or juices as a snack during the long mornings of tennis seemed to decrease the frequency of the attacks, but didn't eliminate them entirely.

In 1969 Sterling's physician had suspected hypoglycemia and had given him a test known as the glucose tolerance test. In fact, over the ensuing eleven years he had put Sterling through *seven* such tests. He concluded on the basis of these tests that Mr. Majors had "reactive hypoglycemia," and prescribed a low-carbohydrate, high-protein diet, with extra snacks during exercise. Because these measures did not fully relieve his symptoms, Sterling attended a lecture on hypoglycemia sponsored by the health education department of a local hospital. The lecturer explained that the glucose tolerance test is totally unreliable as a means of diagnosing hypoglycemia. Sterling thus began to doubt the diagnosis he had been given, and he sought consultation with a specialist in endocrinology and metabolism.

At our first visit Mr. Majors and I agreed that the question of whether he had hypoglycemia could be answered best by measuring his blood sugar levels during his symptoms of weakness and faintness. Fortunately the laboratory associated with my office was open on Saturdays and was not far from the tennis courts where Sterling served, smashed, and volleyed away his happy weekend mornings.

I asked Mr. Majors to get an early start on his tennis games the next Saturday, to skip his usual high-protein snacks during the morning, and to arrange transportation to my office as soon as his symptoms hit him. If the symptoms didn't occur, he was to come to the office after five hours of tennis. I wanted to measure his blood sugar, and examine him, when his symptoms were occurring, or when they were about to begin.

That Saturday he came in around noon, sweaty and tired as one would expect after a long morning of tennis, but he didn't feel faint or ill. His blood sugar was normal, at 73 mg/dl, and his electrocardiogram was normal. I found nothing abnormal on his physical examination, and, although tired, he looked quite fit.

Three weeks later Sterling had one of his faintness attacks halfway through his fourth set of doubles. His partner drove him to my office, conscious but feeling weak, stretched out in the back seat of the car. Physical examination at that time showed a rapid, irregular heartbeat, a low blood pressure, and sweaty, pale skin. His blood sugar was normal at 79 mg/dl. His electrocardiogram was repeated; this time it revealed an abnormality known as paroxysmal atrial fibrillation, or PAF.

His problem was PAF, not hypoglycemia. Low-carbohydrate diets, high-carbohydrate diets, you-name-it kinds of diets don't help PAF. I referred Mr. Majors to a cardiologist, who discovered the cause of his PAF and prescribed the appropriate medications, which are now controlling and preventing the symptoms. He is feeling better now, on appropriate therapy for the condition he actually has. His symptoms never were due to hypoglycemia, even though he carried the diagnosis, and endured the treatment, for thirteen years.

The lesson is clear. Hypoglycemia cannot be diagnosed from your symptoms alone. Questionnaires about your sex life, how you respond to stress, how hungry you get before meals, or how you respond to various foods cannot tell you what your blood sugar is. Neither can hypoglycemia be diagnosed by measuring chemical components of your hair clippings—any more than an empty gas tank can be diagnosed by analyzing paint chips from the roof of your car.

Failure to observe the obvious truism that you must measure the blood sugar during symptoms in order to diagnose hypoglycemia can mislead you and your doctor into treatment for a condition you don't even have. If you do have hypoglycemia, however, then you must find out why your blood sugar is low, so that an intelligent treatment can be pursued.

SUMMARY

1. To find out whether your symptoms are due to low blood sugar, your blood sugar must be measured during the symptoms.
2. If your blood glucose is normal during the symptoms, hypoglycemia is not the cause of those symptoms.
3. If the blood glucose is borderline or definitely low during symptoms, and if the symptoms disappear promptly when the blood sugar is raised, hypoglycemia may well be the cause of your symptoms.
4. People who have never been shown to have low blood sugar during their day-to-day symptoms would do well to question whether they really have hypoglycemia.
5. Unfortunately, the logical first steps outlined above have too often been bypassed, with physicians either assuming that the symptoms are due to hypoglycemia without ever even measuring the blood sugar, or else going on to other procedures such as the oral glucose tolerance test before establishing whether the patient's symptoms have any relationship to his blood sugar.

There are few tests more misunderstood and more likely to mislead both physician and patient than the glucose tolerance test. It has unfortunately become part and parcel of the initial evaluation for hypoglycemia in medical practice throughout this country. We shall therefore spend the next chapter examining this test in detail.

5

Beware the Glucose Tolerance Test

The oral glucose tolerance test (OGTT) was originally devised as a means of studying *high* blood sugar. Unfortunately, the test has become widespread as a means to determine whether someone has *low* blood sugar. Its frequent and unwarranted use has led to the misdiagnosis of hypoglycemia in thousands of people.

To appreciate what it is like to have an OGTT, and what problems its use can lead to, consider the case of Stella Sharp.

Stella works in computer sales for a high-powered electronics firm in California. She is accustomed to pressure and competition, having been a successful student and champion swimmer. Medals and trophies from collegiate and AAU swim meets fill a display case in her apartment. She enjoys the challenge of selling sophisticated data-processing equipment to businesses, though competition has risen to cutthroat levels since Japanese and new American firms have introduced similar product lines.

Stella often takes clients to lunch, and it was following these business lunches that she gradually became aware of symptoms that had bothered her in milder form for years: perspiration, anxiety, rapid heartbeat, a sudden urge to go to the bathroom, and inability to think as clearly as usual. These symptoms especially bothered her in sales-negotiation sessions after lunch, and sometimes too in the mornings while out visiting clients in their offices. She felt these symptoms were robbing her of her competitive edge, so she decided to see her doctor.

As she explained her symptoms to her doctor, he noted that she drank lots of coffee in the mornings—particularly on weekdays when out visiting business offices. She liked her coffee black, with lots of sugar.

There seemed to be no regular pattern to what she ate for lunch. Neither was there any predictable pattern for when the symptoms would strike. Sometimes she would have no symptoms at all. Other times—often when she needed to be at her most charming and persuasive best—the symptoms disturbed her so much she had to cut short an important meeting.

Her physician wondered whether hypoglycemia might not be playing a role in her problems. He had heard that slightly overweight women—like Stella—were often prone to hypoglycemia. He suggested she eliminate the sugar from her coffee, and he ordered a standard diagnostic procedure: a six-hour oral glucose tolerance test, or OGTT.

Stella followed her doctor's instructions faithfully. Except for water, she ate or drank nothing after supper on Thursday night. Friday morning, still fasting, she presented herself at the hospital laboratory at 7:45 A.M. She felt a little hungry, but otherwise well.

Needles didn't bother her, though it seemed impressive that eight blood samples were to be drawn that day, and extra samples when she felt particularly strong symptoms.

At 8:00 A.M. a laboratory technician drew blood from her left forearm for measurement of the fasting glucose level. Stella then had to drink a bottle of carbonated orange-flavored sugar syrup containing a massive 100 grams of glucose. It tasted sickeningly sweet, and was surprisingly difficult to get down in the allotted five minutes. An intense feeling of nausea welled up in her even before she had finished the bottle.

The man next to her in the waiting room, also having a glucose tolerance test, vomited after finishing his bottle, but the lab technician gave him another. This one he managed to keep down by sipping slowly and walking about.

Thirty minutes later when a lab technician drew blood from Stella's right arm her nausea was starting to subside. The lab technician recorded on a worksheet her symptom of nausea (see Fig. 1).

The nausea had pretty well subsided by one hour into the test, when the technician drew more blood from the left arm. The main symptom then was mild dizziness when Stella stood up.

NAME STELLA SHARP DATE 4/31/82

SAMPLE	TIME	SYMPTOMS	PLASMA GLUCOSE
FASTING	8:00	SLIGHT HUNGER	92 - mg/dl
30 MIN.	8:30	NAUSEA	188 "
1 HR.	9:01	DIZZY	194 "
2 HR	10:00	MENTALLY FUZZY, FATIGUE	163 "
EXTRA SAMPLE	10:40	WEAK, WARM, CLAMMY, HEADACHE	121 "
3 HR.	11:00	HEADACHE - SEVERE	103 "
4 HR.	12:06	FATIGUE, HEADACHE, HUNGER	72 "
5 HR	1:00	HEADACHE, MENTALLY DULL	49 "
6 HR	1:58	HEADACHE, CLAMMY, MENTALLY DULL	69 "

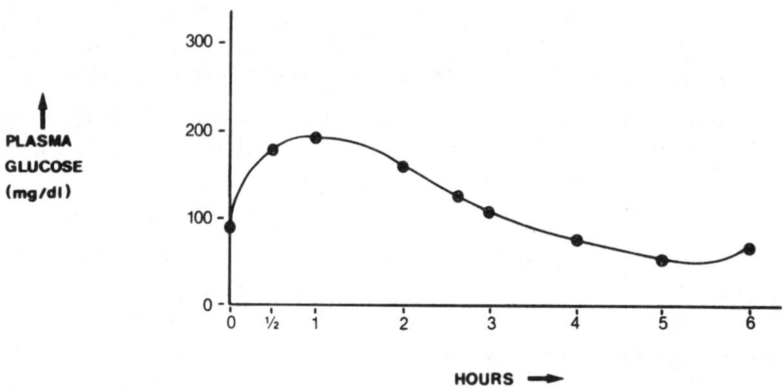

Interpretation: *Mild diabetes with late reactive hypoglycemia*

Ima Slowthinker, M.D.

Fig. 1. Laboratory worksheet for Stella Sharp's first oral glucose tolerance test, with physician's interpretation of the results.

At two hours into the test, when blood was taken from her right arm, Stella felt tired and mentally dull. This was the first symptom that was perhaps similar to what she had experienced on the job, though there was no perspiration, nervousness, or speeding of her heartbeat. A mild headache had begun.

Two hours and 40 minutes into the test she had to move her bowels, and by that time the headache was severe and pounding. She felt weak and hot and clammy. An extra sample of blood was drawn in order to correlate these symptoms with the level of her blood sugar.

The three-hour blood test was accompanied only by the pounding headache, which continued for the rest of the day.

At four hours Stella was starting to feel hungry (it was noon). She was tired, and her head ached. The lab technician had difficulty getting the needle into her vein, but was successful on the third attempt.

Stella's fatigue worsened during the rest of the test, her head continued to throb, and she felt clammy and mentally fuzzy. She had read every magazine in the waiting room, felt she couldn't concentrate, and wanted to lie down.

At 2:00 P.M. the final blood sample was drawn. As she walked out to her car she felt weak and faint, but more than that, she felt she deserved a medal for surviving a modern version of medieval torture.

Instead of a medal, she received a bill for $118 from the hospital laboratory.

Stella's worksheet, with glucose levels filled in, is reproduced in Fig. 1. On the basis of these data, Stella's doctor decided she had a mild and early form of diabetes, in which the blood glucose level rises to abnormal heights, then falls abnormally low. He said she had "the hypoglycemia of early diabetes." He prescribed Diabinese, a drug which lowers blood glucose levels and is widely used in the treatment of mild diabetes mellitus.

Stella went from the doctor's office directly to the library, hoping to read something that would improve her understanding of her predicament. She read that diabetes is a condition in which the blood glucose is too high. As she translated "the hypoglycemia of early diabetes" into her own words, it came out as "the low blood sugar of early high blood sugar." She didn't know whether she was confused or the doctor was confused, but being a reasonable patient she decided to take her pills as prescribed.

While taking a daily 250-mg tablet of chlorpropamide, Stella experienced no improvement in her symptoms. If anything, she felt worse. She put on weight, felt hungry and sweaty at night, and awoke most mornings with a throbbing headache. With this definite deterioration in her condition, Stella became desperate. She stopped taking the chlorpropamide and read a book on hypoglycemia suggested by one of her friends.

The book recommended frequent feedings of low-carbohydrate, high-protein foods. On this diet, and off chlorpropamide, the evening hunger and morning headache subsided, but her original symptoms persisted. She wanted another doctor's opinion, so at the recommendation of a friend she visited the office of an "orthomolecular specialist" who limited his practice to cases of allergy and hypoglycemia.

This "specialist" snipped off a lock of her hair and sent it to Menlo Park, California, for mineral analysis. He also criticized the way in which the previous oral glucose tolerance test had been done, saying that the test was not valid unless preceded by three days of "carbohydrate loading." Stella therefore switched to a high-carbohydrate diet for a few days, then went back to the same hospital lab for a repeat of the same harrowing experience she had been through two months earlier.

This time, however, she was required to produce a urine specimen each time her blood was drawn. With her arms sore and bruised from needle punctures, she reported back to the orthomolecular specialist's office later in the week for analysis of her test results.

The OGTT results, reproduced in Fig. 2, were said to show reactive hypoglycemia. Her blood glucose had fallen to 51 mg/dl three hours into the test. The cause of her reactive hypoglycemia was allegedly revealed by the hair analysis: chromium deficiency, plus weakness of the thyroid and adrenal glands.

Fortunately, the specialist happened to sell the nutritional supplements she would need to correct her deficiencies. Two different types of tablets made from vegetable products fortified with trace minerals would give her the chromium she needed, and extract of beef thyroid and beef adrenal glands would take care of the glandular deficiencies. Her purse bulging with four bottles of pills, she left the specialist's office determined to follow his instructions to the letter. His instructions also included the same

NAME STELLA SHARP DATE 5-30-82

SAMPLE	TIME	SYMPTOMS	PLASMA GLUCOSE
FASTING	8:15	NONE	76 MG/DL
30 MIN.	8:45	NAUSEA	149 "
1 HR.	9:16	MILD NAUSEA	135 "
2 HRS.	10:14	NONE	90 "
3 HRS.	11:15	NONE	51 "
4 HRS.	12:20	FATIGUE	63 "
5 HRS.	1:15	HEADACHE, TIRED, HUNGRY	71 "

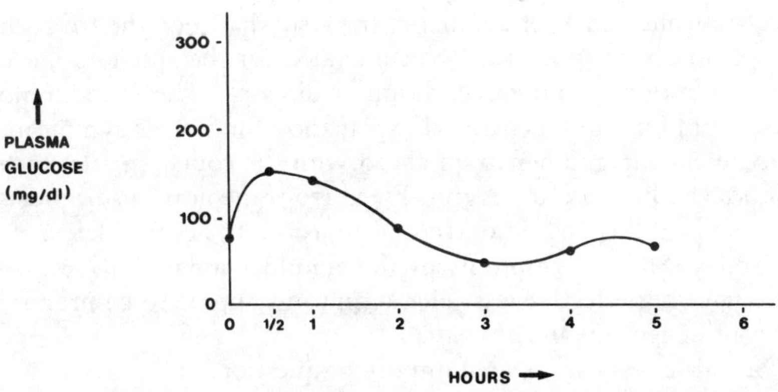

Interpretation:

Reactive hypoglycemia

O.S. Fasttalk, M.D.

Fig. 2. Laboratory worksheet for Stella Sharp's second oral glucose tolerance test, with physician's interpretation of the results.

low-carbohydrate, high-protein, frequent-feeding diet she had read about in the book.

Still the symptoms plagued her—to the point that her sales production began to slip. This led to interviews with her employment supervisor, in whom she confided her problems. Stella was such an outstanding employee that her supervisor tried to help her rather than have her transferred. The supervisor asked the company physician for an opinion, and he recommended consultation with an endocrinologist. The supervisor also recommended a special sales-techniques course to be paid for by the company's career-development fund.

The endocrinologist evaluated Stella's case along the lines suggested in the last chapter. The evaluation showed clearly that her symptoms bore no relation to blood glucose levels. Moreover, the endocrinologist pointed out that both of her glucose tolerance tests had yielded results that were perfectly normal. He also read to her the following inscription in fine print on the bottles of beef-thyroid and beef-adrenal extract she had bought from the orthomolecular specialist: "Not intended for the amelioration or treatment of any known condition or disease." The endocrinologist could find no biochemical explanation for Stella's symptoms, and he encouraged her to go ahead with the course in sales techniques she had already begun. Freed from medical misdiagnosis, she pursued this "common-sense" approach to her problems.

Today, Stella's symptoms are much milder and no longer interfere with her effectiveness. Her symptoms appear to be products of routine tension and anxiety.

Stella's case raises several important questions:

1. Is the OGTT a rational approach to the diagnosis of hypoglycemia?
2. Is there any rational use for a glucose tolerance test?
3. Are there modifications of the OGTT that would make it more useful?
4. How low does the blood glucose go in normal people during an oral glucose tolerance test?
5. How reproducible are the results of OGTTs?
6. What is the significance of symptoms experienced during an OGTT?
7. Does hypoglycemia really lead to diabetes?

The remainder of this chapter will address these questions.

NAME *WILLIE B. WISER* DATE *1982*

SAMPLE	DATE	SYMPTOMS	BANK BALANCE
BASELINE	4/1/82	SHABBY CLOTHES, LONG HAIR, THIN	237.82
½ MONTH	4/15	INEBRIATED	10,237.82
1 "	5/1	GRADES SLIPPING, NEW FRIENDS	9,485.01
1½ "	5/15	SPORTSCAR, CLOTHES BETTER	4,108.90
2 "	6/1	SUDDEN INTEREST IN STOCK MARKET	2,983.66
3 "	7/1	STILL THIN, CLOTHES ? BETTER	674.23
4 "	8/1	GRADES IMPROVING, HAIR LONG	117.04
5 "	9/1	LONESOME	65.98
6 "	10/1	NONE	358.70
7 "	11/1	CLOTHES SHABBY, THIN, HAIR LONG	367.19

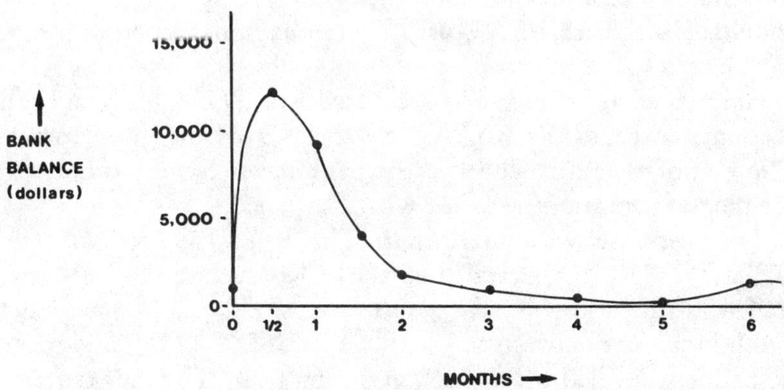

Interpretation:

Mild brief affluence with early reactive hypoprosperity.

Grandpa H.

Fig. 3. Laboratory worksheet for college student's money tolerance test, with interpretation of results by his wealthy grandfather.

Is the glucose tolerance test a rational approach to making the diagnosis of hypoglycemia?

The answer is *no*.

If you want to find out whether the blood sugar is low, *measure* the blood sugar during the symptoms that make you suspect hypoglycemia in the first place. Don't put the patient through the misery of drinking 50 to 100 grams of glucose.

To appreciate how illogical it is to use glucose tolerance testing for the diagnosis of *low blood sugar,* consider the analogous situation of testing for a *low bank account.*

Suppose the grandparents of a college student notice certain symptoms that make them suspect their grandson is out of money: His clothes are old and tattered, he is underweight, and he hasn't had a haircut in almost a year.

What do you think the grandfather should do to find out whether his grandson is broke? Should he check the balance in his grandson's account (measure the money level)? Of course he should. Instead, this hypothetical grandfather devised a "money tolerance test."

Here is what he did. He deposited $10,000 in his grandson's account, and had the bank notify the boy of his good fortune. The grandfather then checked the bank balance every other week for the next six months to see what happened.

The response was interesting. The bank balance rose from $237.82 to $10,237.82 and then started to decline. The grandson traded in his motorbike for a sportscar, and bought some stocks and bonds. The account fell to a low of $65.98 at the five-month point, then leveled off at $360 at six months. The hair remained uncut, the clothes improved marginally, and the boy put on a few pounds. The results looked impressive when compiled in graphic form, as shown in Fig. 3, but the grandfather was left to wonder what he had learned from his "scientific" experiment. What he had learned was how his progeny tended to dispose of excess funds.

You can indeed find out something about someone's financial "money metabolism" by putting an extra $10,000 into his account. It may help you diagnose certain problems in his or her financial management, such as a tendency to gamble or an allergy to saving money. But it does not tell you whether or not the person is broke. Once you already know he is broke, a money tolerance test may help you find out how he got that way, but as a means of finding out *whether* he is broke, it is illogical and unnecessary.

In the same way that a money tolerance test has little bearing on a person's day-to-day finances, an oral glucose tolerance test has little bearing on everyday energy metabolism. The oral glucose tolerance test is an unnatural and artificial stress. A breakfast of 50–100 grams of pure glucose is not a normal meal, even in modern America. What happens to your blood sugar after such a metabolic insult is practically irrelevant to the symptoms experienced by people in ordinary day-to-day life.

You don't diagnose poverty by handing out checks for $10,000, and you don't diagnose hypoglycemia by pouring 100 grams of glucose into someone's stomach—even though the experience is sure to be a memorable one.

The proper way to diagnose hypoglycemia is to measure the blood glucose during the symptoms that under normal circumstances suggest low blood sugar. Once you know the blood sugar *is* low, a glucose tolerance test *may* help you find out how it became low, but like the money tolerance test, it is seldom necessary.

Is there any rational use for a glucose tolerance test?

The answer is *yes*.

The oral glucose tolerance test (OGTT) is useful in the diagnosis of an unusual disease caused by a tumor of the pituitary gland that overproduces growth hormone. For example, a patient of mine had *high* blood sugar because of just such a tumor. The excess growth hormone was driving her blood sugar upward. We did a one-hour glucose tolerance test to prove that her secretion of growth hormone was abnormal. As her blood sugar rose after the glucose drink, her growth-hormone level did not fall as it would in a normal person. The test helped clinch the diagnosis of a growth-hormone-secreting tumor of the pituitary. Surgery to remove the tumor brought the growth-hormone levels back down to normal, and cured the high blood sugar.

Since the glucose tolerance test ordinarily induces an initial rise in blood sugar, it also causes a rise in insulin secretion and a fall in growth-hormone secretion in healthy persons. The OGTT can be used, therefore, to study disorders of the secretion of these two hormones. Its main use has been as a *research* tool for the investigation of diabetes mellitus, in which blood glucose levels are high, and rise abnormally higher after sugar is eaten. Unfortunately, even as a test for diabetes the OGTT has been greatly misinterpreted. This is because the levels of blood glucose defined as abnormally high, or "diabetic," were originally set too low, and have only recently been revised.[1] The result has been that many people, like Stella, have been mistakenly told they have mild diabetes. Moreover, in actual practice, the fasting level of blood glucose is almost always sufficient to diagnose diabetes,[2] so that the OGTT is seldom necessary.

In the evaluation of hypoglycemia, an OGTT may occasionally be helpful. For example, persons with hypoglycemia that is due to abnormally rapid emptying of the stomach may show a characteristic pattern of blood sugar levels on an OGTT. They demonstrate a rapid extreme rise in blood glucose following the oral glucose drink, and then a precipitous fall to abnormally low levels. Before applying the OGTT to such a case, however, one would logically *first* show that low blood sugar occurs following the meals normally eaten by that person.

The story of an exceptional patient, with unusual dietary practices, was related by Dr. Leonard Madison, a professor of medicine and endocrinology who has done much to bring reason and clarity to the subject of hypoglycemia. This patient loved waffles for breakfast. An hour or two after breakfast the patient often had symptoms suggestive of low blood sugar. When the patient explained his history in detail, he disclosed that he ate his waffles in a big cereal bowl. The cereal bowl held more syrup than a plate, and what that man *really* liked to eat was syrup. He was essentially having a glucose tolerance test every morning for breakfast! Hypoglycemia was being induced by bizarre eating habits. In this case, the OGTT confirmed what had been found following one of his soggy-waffle breakfasts: The blood sugar rose rapidly, then fell very low with hypoglycemic symptoms as the result.

Are there modifications of the OGTT that would make it more useful?

The answer is that oral glucose tolerance tests are seldom needed in the first place, apart from research, but that yes, certain

[1] National Diabetes Data Group, *Diabetes* 28 (1979), 1039.

[2] A fasting level of 140 mg/dl, repeated at least once, is now generally accepted as adequate evidence of diabetes mellitus.

modifications from the usual procedure may increase the value of the test in specific cases. Unfortunately, as in the case of Stella, OGTTs are frequently repeated, with modifications, when the test isn't necessary in the first place.

A common addition to the OGTT is the measurement of urine glucose levels simultaneous with the blood measurements. This indicates the level of blood glucose that must be attained before a person's kidneys allow glucose to escape from the blood into the urine. This information may be helpful in *treating* diabetes, but it is useless in trying to make the *diagnosis* of either hypoglycemia or diabetes. Moreover, the pathological condition in which glucose escapes into the urine at normal blood glucose levels (known as "renal glycosuria") does not cause hypoglycemia. Thus, this addition to the OGTT has no place in the intelligent evaluation of hypoglycemia.

A much more expensive addition to the OGTT is the measurement of blood levels of insulin. Insulin levels do rise during an OGTT, but these levels do not help determine whether the patient has abnormally low blood sugar. Only *after* one has shown that the patient has hypoglycemia is it useful to measure insulin levels, and even then it's not helpful to measure insulin levels *during* the OGTT. The pattern of insulin secretion during the OGTT has been carefully studied in a scientific manner, and shows no correlation with the pattern of blood glucose response.[3,4] The intelligent use of insulin measurement in discovering why someone has hypoglycemia will be discussed in Chapter 9; it does not involve glucose tolerance testing.

Another "twist," or modification, in the OGTT involves dietary preparation. The amount of carbohydrate eaten for a few days prior to glucose tolerance testing influences how high and how low the blood sugar will go, and how much insulin will be secreted during the OGTT, but still does not render the test relevant or useful in evaluating the possibility of hypoglycemia.

The most logical and useful modification of the oral glucose tolerance test has been to dispense with the bottle of sugar syrup entirely, and to conduct instead a "breakfast tolerance test." In this test, a standard meal of regular food is eaten, and the blood glucose response is measured. This removes much of the artificiality of glucose tolerance testing, and better imitates the normal

[3] **A. S. Luyckx and P. J. Lefebvre, *Diabetes* 20 (1971), 435.**
[4] **F. D. Hofeldt et al., *Diabetes* 23 (1974), 589**

day-to-day situation. Since it is the daily situation of the patient that needs to be investigated, however, the logical first step remains as outlined in Chapter 4: Have the patient eat his usual breakfast or lunch, or hot fudge sundae, or whatever it is that precipitates symptoms, and then measure the blood glucose level during the outbreak of the symptoms. *After* this procedure has demonstrated hypoglycemia, *then* the breakfast tolerance test makes sense as a way to distinguish between abnormal eating habits (as with the patient who ate syrup for breakfast) and abnormal metabolism.

How low does the blood glucose go in normal people during an OGTT?

This is an important question, because thousands of people have been put through oral glucose tolerance tests and have been told on the basis of the results that they have hypoglycemia. Even though the OGTT is an unnatural provocation and irrelevant to most people's daily symptoms, these people need to know whether their results are truly abnormal. Fortunately, some excellent medical research has addressed this problem.

Medical scientists in Boston, led by Dr. B. N. Park and Dr. J. S. Soeldner,[5] performed five-hour OGTTs on 123 *normal* persons. Of these normal people, 23% had blood glucose levels *under* 50 mg/dl during the test. Remember, these were people who did *not* have day-to-day symptoms of hypoglycemia. They took the OGTT only because someone paid them to do it for research purposes, yet nearly *one-fourth* of them had blood sugar levels low enough to be labeled as hypoglycemic by many physicians.

The logical conclusion to reach from this study is that blood glucose levels under 50 mg/dl *during an OGTT* are not necessarily abnormal, and do not signify disease.

I emphasize these figures because in my experience most people who have been diagnosed hypoglycemic on the basis of glucose tolerance tests have had normal blood glucose patterns. Their doctors, however, have interpreted levels in the 40s and 50s as abnormal, and diagnostic of hypoglycemia. Research results refute the notion that such levels are abnormal.

An even more detailed study was carried out in the University of Missouri School of Medicine by Dr. T. W. Burns and col-

[5] B. N. Park et al., *Diabetes* 21 (Suppl. 21, 1972), 373.

leagues.[6] They measured blood glucose continuously (not just every 30–60 minutes) during five-hour OGTTs in 28 healthy, normal adults. These were men and women between the ages of 17 and 42 years, who had no symptoms of hypoglycemia. Of the 28 normal subjects, one achieved a blood glucose as low as 30 mg/dl, another reached 34 mg/dl, and three others went as low as 40 mg/dl. Nine of the 28 subjects had blood sugars of 50 mg/dl or lower at some time during the test. In other words, by measuring the blood glucose continuously, instead of intermittently, the researchers showed that 32% of these normal subjects dropped their blood glucose levels to 50 mg/dl or lower.

Since one-third of normal people have blood glucose levels as low as 50 mg/dl during oral glucose tolerance testing, the logical conclusion is that *this is one of the normal patterns of response* to the unnatural stimulus of an OGTT. Another logical way of looking at it is to conclude that a "meal" of 100 grams of glucose, taken on an empty stomach, can be *normally* expected to cause the blood glucose to fall (usually after an initial rise), and that in about one-third of normal persons this fall will be to 50 mg/dl or less.

Dr. Burns carried out a similar experiment with himself as part of a group of 12 normal human volunteers, and found that within that group *42%* had blood glucose levels *under* 50 mg/dl during the OGTT.[7] His own level fell to 48 mg/dl at three hours and 23 minutes into the test. Now if he had not been continuously measuring the blood glucose and had instead taken samples hourly, he would have missed this low point. These studies show that how low a level you get during an OGTT depends on when you happen to take the blood sample. Intermittent sampling, in face of continuous variation of blood glucose levels, will produce variable results. This is part of the reason why normal people, like Stella, can have such variable results from one OGTT to the next.

How reproducible are the results of oral glucose tolerance tests?

The answer is, *not very*.

Remember the case of Sterling Majors, recounted in Chapter 4. He was the man who had a heart problem (PAF) that made him feel very faint and weak when it occurred typically during tennis matches on Saturday mornings. For thirteen years he was misdi-

[6] **T. W. Burns et al., *Journal of Laboratory and Clinical Medicine* 65 (1965), 927.**
[7] **T. W. Burns et al., *Diabetes* 14 (1965), 186.**

Table 1

ORAL GLUCOSE TOLERANCE TEST RESULTS IN STERLING MAJORS, 1969–1982

Date	*Fasting*	*½ Hour*	*1 Hour*	*2 Hours*	*3 Hours*	*4 Hours*	*5 Hours*	*Symptoms during the test as recorded by the laboratory technician*
11/3/69	96	190	192	150	68	86	95	3 hours—patient complained of light-headedness. 4–5 hours—patient lay down, still felt somewhat light-headed but all right.
10/13/71	68	171	194	157	81	64	65	Patient became dizzy and lay down between 3–4 hours.
3/12/73	85	218	224	150	41	70	79	3 hours—patient shaky, dizzy, lay down.
1/17/75	100	220	240	183	70	80	80	5 hours—very faint.
1/7/76	82	—	140	95	62	71	85	Patient slightly dizzy 3–4 hours. No other symptoms.
4/18/79	90	194	169	98	42	59	72	Felt fine until 4 hours, 5 hours, when felt light-headed.
3/3/82	85	184	157	106	39	71	81	(No entry by lab technician on this test report.)

agnosed as having hypoglycemia on the basis of oral glucose tolerance tests. The actual laboratory results of the seven OGTTs he endured are shown in Table 1.

All of his glucose tolerance tests results are normal, yet they vary greatly from one test to the next. The tests done in 1969, 1971, 1973, and 1975 would be misinterpreted by some physicians as showing mild diabetes mellitus. The tests of 1973, 1979, and 1982 would be misinterpreted by many as showing hypoglycemia. As a matter of fact, Sterling Majors's glucose metabolism has been normal all along. His responses to the unnatural stress of an oral glucose tolerance test show how unpredictable and unreproducible the results of this test are in normal people.

Sterling Majors is not the only person with normal glucose metabolism to undergo repeated oral glucose tolerance tests. In 1965 a group of medical researchers led by Dr. G. W. McDonald carefully conducted glucose tolerance tests on more than 400 inmates at a federal prison.[8] These were healthy "volunteers." Each of the 400 prisoners took a three-hour OGTT every two months for a year. Each prisoner thus went through six different OGTTs, and Dr. McDonald evaluated how much variation occurred from one test to another in the same individual. The results were discouraging, to say the least. He reported that a "wide range of variability was found at all glucose levels in this population of nondiabetic men." It was typical for a man's test result at a given point in the OGTT to vary as much as plus or minus 34 mg/dl from one test to another. For example, the value at one hour after the glucose drink might be 100 mg/dl on one occasion, 134 mg/dl on the next, and 66 mg/dl on the next. Approximately 20% of the inmates varied even more than this.

How can you base a diagnosis on a test that varies so much from one test to another in the same individual? Not very well. Dr. McDonald lamented, "With variations of this magnitude . . . it is difficult to interpret, with any degree of confidence, single glucose tolerance tests that show abnormalities which are not extreme. It was possible, and it did occur in our population, for a man to vary from normal readings to those considered abnormal over several tests." The researchers summarized their results by writing that "these data do not support reproducibility of numerical values or of positive or diagnostic test results."

[8] G. W. McDonald, G. H. Fisher, and C. Burnham, *Diabetes* 14 (1965), 473.

A follow-up study by some of the same research team compared four different OGTTs in each of 96 young healthy prison inmates.[9] In two of the OGTTs, 50 grams of glucose were given, and in the other two 100 grams were given. In no case could they show a reliable degree of reproducibility for the OGTT. They concluded, "The fact that only a moderate degree of correlation was found between repeat tolerance responses greatly compromises the clinical value of a single glucose tolerance test."

One more note on this carefully conducted research in healthy men: 30% of them had blood glucose values measured at 50 mg/dl or below, even though only three samples of blood were taken after the glucose drink during each OGTT—showing again that low levels of blood sugar are normal during an OGTT and are not indicative of disease.

What is the significance of symptoms experienced during an OGTT?

The answer is twofold.

First, the symptoms are irrelevant to the patient's usual symptoms unless the patient usually eats huge quantities of sugar on an empty stomach. We have already reviewed in Chapter 2 the general principle that the same symptoms can arise from different causes. Consequently, just because you have symptoms during an OGTT that resemble those in daily life doesn't prove that the cause of the symptoms is the same.

Second, symptoms experienced during an OGTT bear little relation to blood glucose levels. This point was underscored by Dr. Vincent Marks, who is a leading scientist in the field of hypoglycemia and holds the position of Professor of Clinical Biochemistry at the University of Surrey in England. Dr. Marks evaluated 65 consecutive patients referred to the Epsom District Hospital for five-hour oral glucose tolerance tests.[10] All of these patients were suspected by their doctors of having abnormal glucose metabolism, such as diabetes or hypoglycemia. The patients were interviewed carefully about symptoms that were suggestive of hypoglycemia. Symptoms that occurred "spontaneously" in

[9] C. W. Sisk et al., *Diabetes* 19 (1970), 852.

[10] V. Marks, "Hypoglycemia: Proceedings of the European Symposium Rome, *Hormone and Metabolic Research* (Suppl. 6) (Stuttgart: Georg Thieme Publishers, 1976), 1.

everyday life were noted, as well as symptoms encountered during the OGTT. Fig. 4 shows the results.

A study of Fig. 4 will corroborate our two-part answer to the question about the meaning of symptoms during an OGTT. First, whether you have symptoms during the OGTT has little to do with whether you had them spontaneously under normal circumstances. Second, whether you have symptoms during an OGTT has little to do with how low your blood sugar goes.

These studies directly refute the notion that oral glucose tolerance tests help clarify whether someone's spontaneous symptoms arise from hypoglycemia. The simple fact is that the OGTT is the wrong test to answer this question. The right test is a measurement of the level of blood glucose during a spontaneous outbreak of the symptoms.

Dr. A. A. Abbasi and his colleagues in Michigan provided a still more elegant demonstration of the lack of relationship between everyday symptoms and blood sugar levels during glucose tolerance testing.[11] They studied seven patients whose blood sugars fell to an average of 45 mg/dl during an OGTT. Each of these seven had spontaneous symptoms in everyday life consistent with hypoglycemia and were diagnosed as having "reactive hypoglycemia." Dr. Abbasi's team then treated all seven patients with a drug, propantheline, that *prevented* the fall in blood sugar during the OGTT. The average low point in the OGTT while taking the drug was 76 mg/dl—nowhere near the hypoglycemic range. Nevertheless, the patients experienced no improvement in daily symptoms while taking the drug for three to twelve months.

A superficially similar study was carried out by Dr. Permutt and his co-workers in St. Louis.[12] They studied seven patients who had symptoms suggestive of hypoglycemia and whose blood glucose level fell to an average low point of 44 mg/dl during OGTTs. Using the same drug that Dr. Abbasi's group had employed, they were also able to prevent the blood glucose from falling during an OGTT. Unfortunately, these scientists did not report whether the drug made the patients feel better in everyday life. The patients' symptoms during the OGTT were improved while taking the propantheline, but, as explained above, symptoms during an OGTT bear little or no relationship to daily life.

[11] A. A. Abbasi et al., *Diabetes* 24 (Suppl. 2, 1975), 425.
[12] M. A. Permutt, D. Keller, and J. Santiago, *Diabetes* 26 (1977), 121.

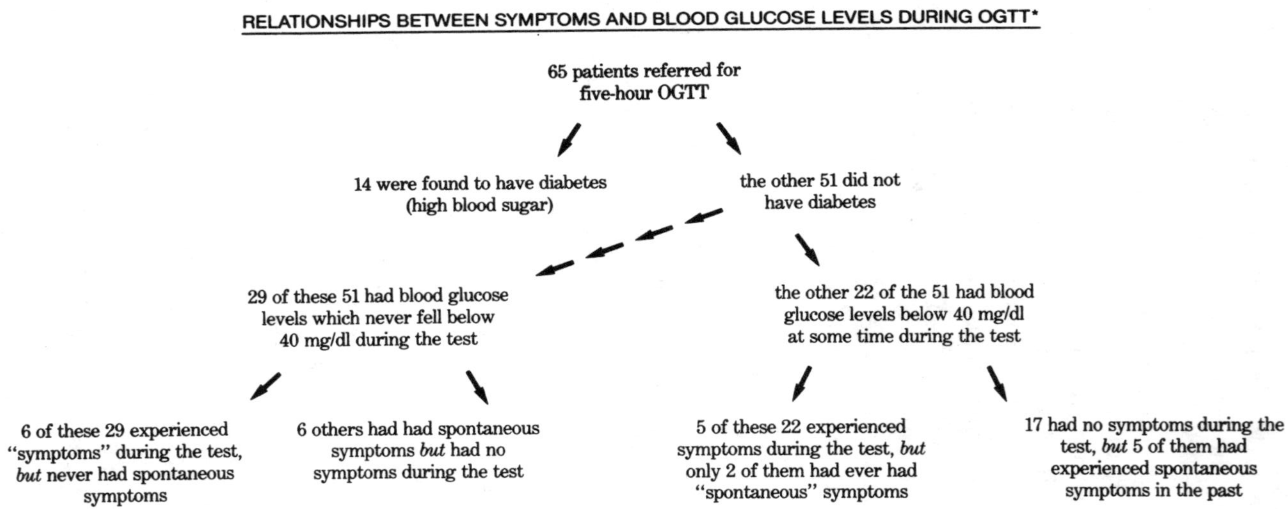

*Marks V: *Hormone & Metabolic Research* (Suppl. 6) "Hypoglycemia: Proceedings of the European Symposium Rome" Georg Thieme Publishers, Stuttgart, pages 1–6, 1976.

Fig. 4. Lack of relationship between blood glucose levels during a 5-hour oral glucose tolerance test (OGTT) and "hypoglycemic" symptoms. There are no clear connections among (1) spontaneous symptoms in daily life, (2) symptoms during the OGTT, and (3) glucose levels during the OGTT. Therefore, the OGTT does not clarify the nature of spontaneous symptoms experienced in daily life. "Hypoglycemic" symptoms can occur during an OGTT regardless of whether similar symptoms occur spontaneously in daily life, and regardless of whether hypoglycemia occurs during the test. *(Used by permission.)*

Despite the thousands of suffering people diagnosed by OGTTs as having reactive hypoglycemia, no convincing data have ever been published to prove that propantheline improves their spontaneous day-to-day symptoms. The fact that the drug makes people feel better during an OGTT is merely further evidence that the OGTT is irrelevant to normal daily living.

Does hypoglycemia really lead to diabetes?

The answer is, *almost never*.

This fact will surprise many people. One of the most widespread myths about hypoglycemia is that it occurs commonly in the early stages of diabetes or is itself an early stage of diabetes. This mistaken notion has arisen from the use of the oral glucose tolerance test (OGTT) to diagnose diabetes and hypoglycemia. In most such cases the OGTT results were misinterpreted, and hypoglycemia and diabetes were misdiagnosed.

Accurately diagnosed cases of actual hypoglycemia which later developed diabetes are rare. A small handful of such cases has been published in scientific journals. For example, drugs or infections that cause diabetes by destroying the insulin-producing cells of the pancreas may briefly liberate excess insulin into the bloodstream, causing temporary hypoglycemia. Such cases are rare. The popular notion, however, has been that this sequence of low, then high, blood sugar occurs in the usual type of diabetes that affects overweight adults. This notion is false.

No data proving that hypoglycemia is a forerunner or early stage of mild, adult-onset diabetes have ever been published. Respectable authors have stated in many articles and textbooks that patients in the early stages of diabetes often go through a phase of hypoglycemia. But published data to prove the point do not exist.

It is one thing to *claim* at the poker table that you are holding a royal flush. It is quite another to prove it by laying your cards face up on the table. In medical research you lay your cards on the table by publishing your data. Until this occurs, the rest of us are entitled to be cautious about believing claims, even those made by authoritative persons.

Although a few patients with documented hypoglycemia have later developed diabetes mellitus, there is no evidence of any greater risk, or likelihood, of diabetes in persons who have had hypoglycemia than in persons who have never had it. Published reports to the contrary are based on definitions of diabetes that have since been discredited.

There is a good explanation for the confusion about the relation, or lack of relation, between hypoglycemia and diabetes. Use of the OGTT has muddled the diagnosis of diabetes mellitus almost as thoroughly as that of hypoglycemia. It used to be thought that a blood glucose greater than 120 mg/dl two hours after the oral load meant diabetes. Now, however, experts agree[13] that the blood glucose must exceed 200 mg/dl at the two-hour point, and that this finding must be confirmed by a repeat test, before diabetes should be diagnosed on the basis of an OGTT. Untold hundreds of people whose two-hour blood sugar on OGTT was over 120 mg/dl, but under 200 mg/dl, have in all likelihood been erroneously diagnosed as having diabetes mellitus. It is this group of "mild diabetics" (actually not diabetic at all) who have been mislabeled as having reactive hypoglycemia because (like other normal people) their blood glucose levels may drop below 50 mg/dl sometime during an OGTT. Stella's case epitomized this problem of double misdiagnosis by OGTT.

If you use incorrect criteria for the diagnosis of diabetes and incorrect criteria for the diagnosis of hypoglycemia, the OGTT will lead you to believe that people shift from one disease to the other. This was the case in the normal, healthy prisoners who underwent repeated OGTTs in the research cited earlier. Some of them, on the basis of their OGTT results, looked diabetic at one time and hypoglycemic at another, *if* you apply outdated criteria for both conditions. In reality, however, these men were neither diabetic nor hypoglycemic. They were healthy. Their responses to the OGTTs merely showed how variable the results of that test can be.

SUMMARY

To summarize the main points of this chapter:

1. The oral glucose tolerance test (OGTT) is an irrational approach to the diagnosis of hypoglycemia and is irrelevant to the everyday symptoms of anyone whose diet does not consist of huge doses of pure sugar.

[13] National Diabetes Data Group. *Diabetes* 28 (1979), 1039.

2. Many of the symptoms experienced during an OGTT are not related to the blood glucose level.
3. The OGTT produces an extremely broad and variable range of blood sugar responses in normal people.
4. Many people have been mistakenly diagnosed as having hypoglycemia on the basis of an OGTT.
5. Many people have been mistakenly diagnosed as having diabetes mellitus on the basis of an OGTT.
6. There is no firm evidence that hypoglycemia is a forerunner or early stage of diabetes.

Having spent a chapter contending with popular misconceptions about abnormal blood sugar metabolism, let's now turn our attention to the normal functioning of the human body. Understanding how the body controls blood sugar will serve as a foundation for understanding what can go wrong and cause hypoglycemia.

6

What Controls the Level of Blood Sugar?

The level of glucose in the blood, like the level of water in a river, is determined by the balance of input and outflow. Water flows into a river from incoming streams, from rainfall, and from snow melting on its banks. Water leaves a river through outflowing streams, evaporation, and seepage into the ground. The exact level of water in the river is the balanced result of these opposing processes. A river can run dry because of abnormally low input (as during a drought), or because of excessively rapid outflow. So it is with the level of blood sugar.

Sugar flows *into* the bloodstream from three sources: (1) absorption of food, (2) liberation of glucose from the breakdown of animal starch (glycogen), and (3) the production of new sugar within the body (gluconeogenesis).

Sugar flows *out* of the bloodstream by entering into body tissues. The blood, after all, is simply a transportation system that carries nutrients (such as sugar, fat, and protein) and oxygen to the tissues of the body, and picks up waste products (such as carbon dioxide and urea) to be transported to the lungs and kidneys for disposal. In normal people, no significant amount of sugar is lost into sweat, urine, or breath. It all goes from the blood into various body tissues.

In a 24-hour period, all of these normal processes of glucose input and outflow occur in healthy people. To understand them better, let's follow the path of a baked potato as it is eaten for dinner. Please see Fig. 5.

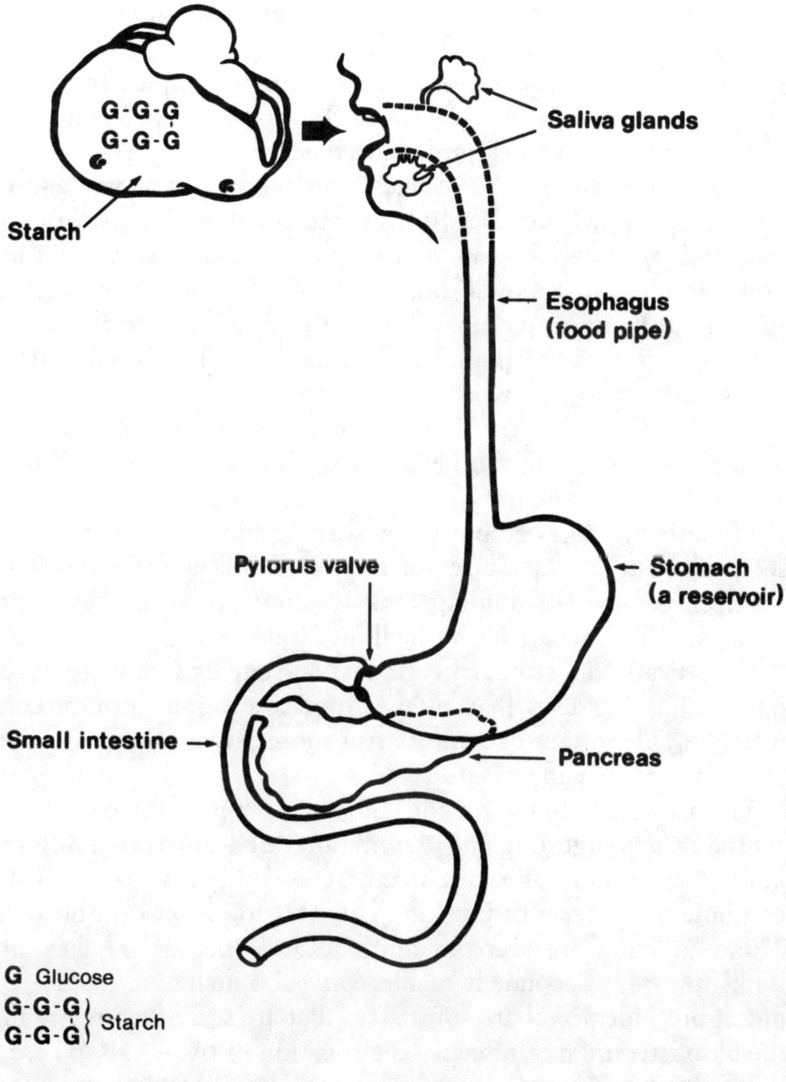

Fig. 5. A baked potato with sour cream, about to be eaten. The starch in the potato is made of glucose. Once the starch is broken down into individual glucose molecules, these will enter the bloodstream, raising the level of blood glucose.

Potatoes are composed largely of starch, which is made up of many glucose molecules chained together. This starch has to be broken down into individual glucose molecules before it can be absorbed. The process of breaking down complex foods (like starch and protein) into their simple building blocks (such as glucose and amino acids) is termed *digestion*.

Even before the potato reaches your mouth, its aroma and the idea of eating it have already triggered the digestive process. Saliva starts to flow, the pancreas may begin to secrete insulin into your bloodstream. As you chew and roll the first bite of potato in your mouth, digestive enzymes in the saliva attack the starch, splitting off individual glucose molecules. That is why starch tastes sweet if you chew it long enough.

Swallowing sends the bite of potato down to your stomach, where acid attacks it and helps break it down into still simpler, absorbable components. The stomach acts as a reservoir, holding the food being digested but not absorbing much of it. As we shall see later, one of the causes of hypoglycemia is a failure of the stomach to act as a holding tank to slow down the absorption process, which occurs in the small intestine.

Periodically the stomach contracts and the exit valve (pylorus) opens, allowing a small amount of food to progress into the small intestine. There the food meets still more powerful digestive enzymes from the pancreas.

The pancreas, lying behind and below the stomach, plays a central role in digesting and assimilating food. It has two different kinds of secretions. First, it manufactures digestive *enzymes* that continue the process of breaking complex foods into simple ones. These enzymes are secreted into the intestine, where they mix with the food. Second, it makes *hormones,* including insulin and glucagon. Hormones are substances that are secreted directly into the bloodstream and influence the function of tissues elsewhere in the body. Insulin and glucagon influence the handling of glucose by many tissues throughout the body, including liver, fat, and muscle.

Specialized nests of cells within the pancreas produce the hormones insulin and glucagon. These nests are named "islets of Langerhans," after their discoverer. Fig. 6 diagrams the location of these special cells, as well as the sources of other hormones

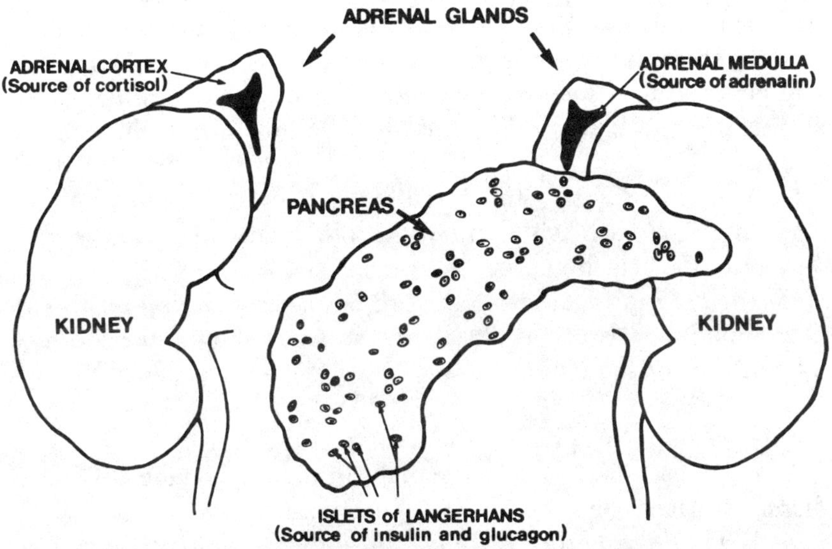

Fig. 6. Sources of several hormones important in human glucose metabolism. Cortisol comes from the outer portion of the adrenal gland, known as the adrenal cortex. The center portion of the adrenal gland (adrenal medulla) makes adrenalin, or epinephrine. Insulin and glucagon come from specialized cells within the islets of Langerhans of the pancreas.

important in glucose metabolism. We'll discuss the other hormones later.

The pancreas secretes insulin into the bloodstream in response to at least three signals. First, the nervous system notifies the pancreas that food is about to be eaten and absorbed. Second, during absorption the rising level of glucose and other nutrients in the blood triggers insulin release. Third, other hormones secreted from the intestine stimulate the pancreas to secrete even more insulin. These "insulin-boosting" hormones are made in the intestinal wall, and are secreted when food arrives from the stomach. As we shall see in coming chapters, these hormones involved in the control of glucose metabolism play a role in several causes of hypoglycemia.

As food leaves the stomach and enters the intestine, several important processes go forward at once in a beautifully coordinated fashion. Hormones are released from the intestine to boost insulin secretion in the pancreas, and other hormones stimulate the pancreas to deliver digestive enzymes into the intestine. These pancreatic enzymes break the food down into simple, absorbable components. Lining the walls of the small intestine are other digestive enzymes that finish the job of breaking down complex carbohydrates such as starch into simple sugars, like glucose, that can enter the cells lining the intestine.

From the intestinal cells, glucose passes into the bloodstream. The blood vessels that drain the intestine, as shown in Fig. 7, go directly to the liver. On the way, insulin from the pancreas joins the glucose.

The insulin "programs" the liver and the rest of the body to take up the sugar. It is like a signal to the body saying, "Food is here. Nutrients are abundant. Open up and let them into your cells." Thus the body, working through the pancreas, sets into motion the *outflow* of glucose from the blood into the tissues at the same time that glucose flows into the bloodstream from the intestine. This close coordination between outflow and inflow prevents the blood sugar from going too high or too low.

Now let's look at the main character in this metabolic drama—the liver. Fig. 7 shows that all glucose absorbed through the intestine goes directly to the liver. The largest organ in the body, the liver acts as a central clearinghouse for glucose. It receives all glucose absorbed from the intestines. It stores glucose in the form of glycogen, or "animal starch," similar to the vegetable starch found in potatoes. It exports glucose to the rest of the body as needed to supply energy and maintain a normal blood glucose level. The liver also manufactures *new* glucose from amino acids. The liver thus plays a central role in maintaining a normal blood glucose level. A sick liver can obviously be a cause of low blood sugar.

The liver acts on glucose under the influence of several hormones, especially insulin and glucagon flowing in from the pancreas. The wrong amount or wrong timing of these hormones can cause hypogylcemia, as we shall see in the next two chapters.

Fig. 8 depicts the glucose from our potato as it arrives in the liver. The glucose molecules enter freely into the liver cells. Insu-

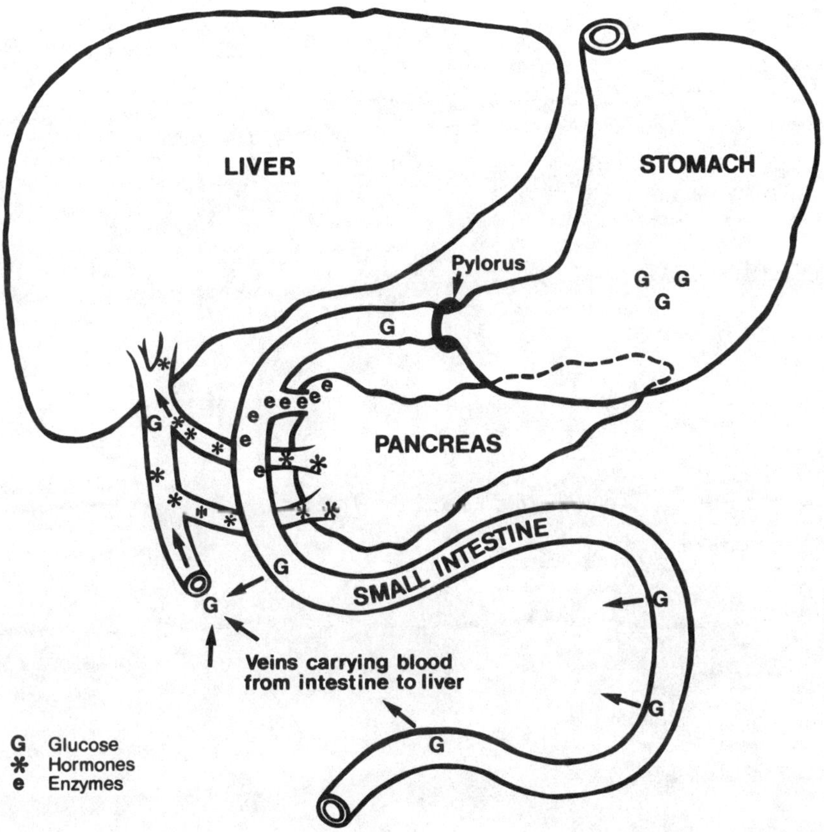

Fig. 7. The pancreas secretes digestive enzymes into the intestine, where they help break food down into simple, absorbable molecules such as glucose. The intestine then absorbs glucose into the bloodstream, which carries the glucose directly to the liver. Meanwhile, the pancreas secretes insulin into the blood vessels that lead to the liver.

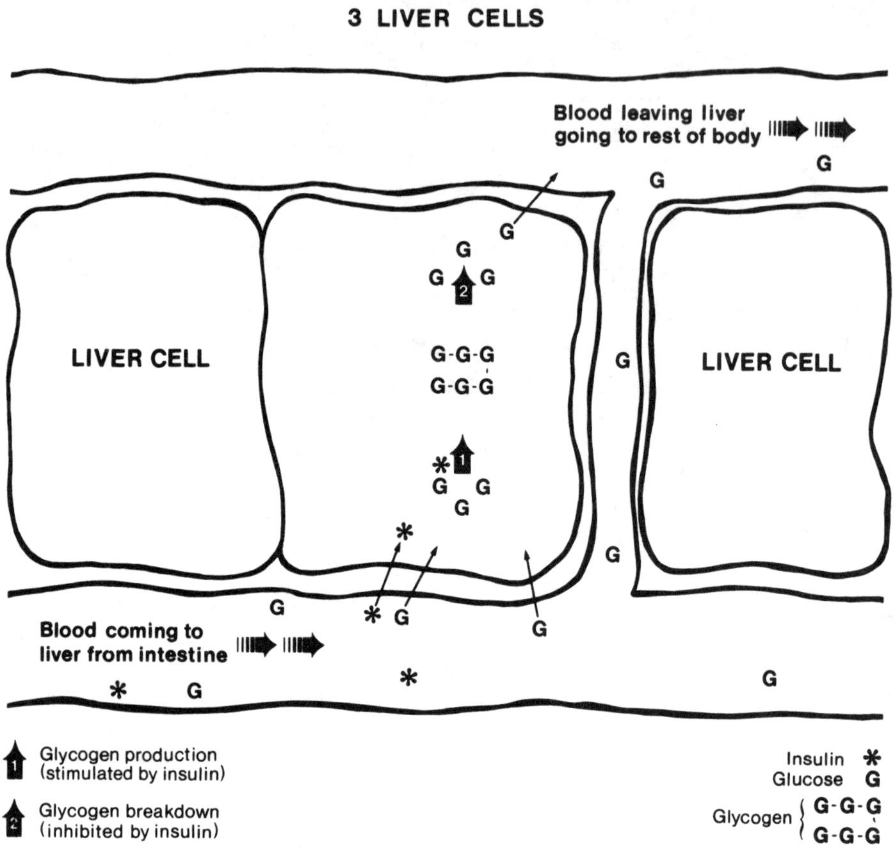

Fig. 8. Within the liver, glucose enters cells and is stored as glycogen. Insulin activates liver-cell enzymes to produce glycogen from the glucose. Lack of insulin favors glycogen breakdown, resulting in the release of glucose from the liver into the bloodstream. Glucagon and epinephrine also promote glycogen breakdown, and thereby raise the level of blood glucose.

lin has already set in motion the liver-cell machinery that chains some of the glucose together for storage as *glycogen*. Similar to vegetable starch, glycogen consists of chains of glucose molecules bonded together. Not all of the glucose from the potato will go into glycogen. Some slips through the liver and is available immediately for the energy needs of the brain and other tissues.

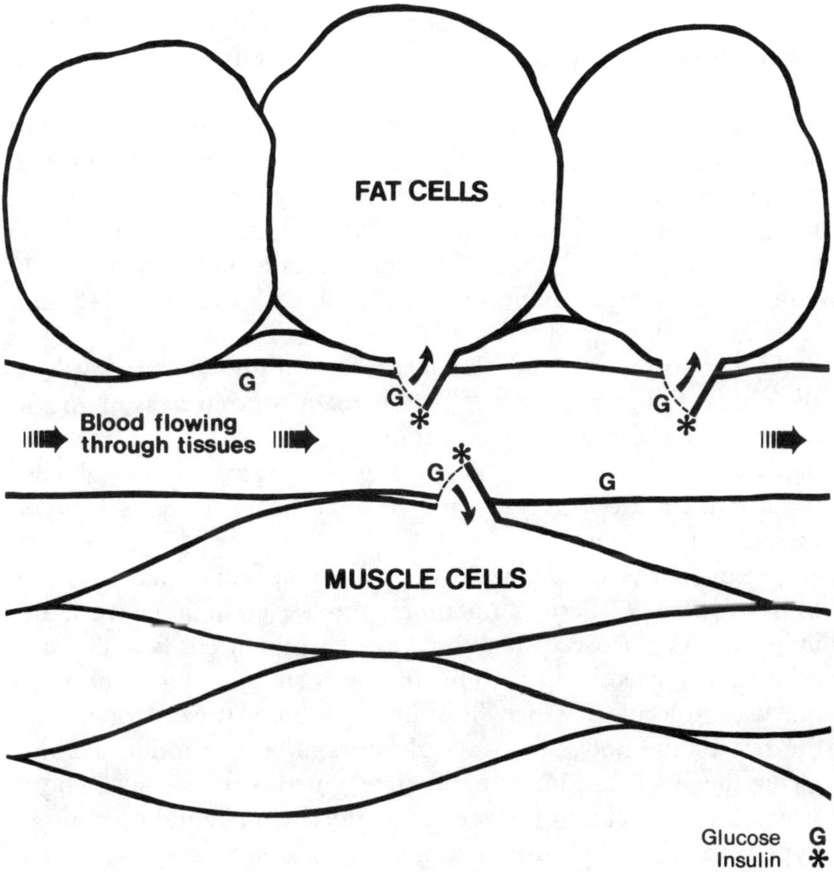

Fig. 9. Insulin acts on fat and muscle cells to facilitate the uptake of glucose from the bloodstream. In this way, insulin accelerates glucose outflow from the bloodstream and lowers the level of blood sugar.

The glucose molecules that have slipped on through the liver can be taken up into the brain or other tissues. The insulin in the blood signals the tissues that this extra glucose is available and should be taken up. As shown in Fig. 9 some of the glucose enters fat cells and is incorporated into fat. Other glucose enters muscle cells and is either consumed as fuel or stored as glycogen within the muscle.

The potato, representing about 25,000 milligrams of glucose, has now been disposed of along with the sour cream, broccoli, hollandaise sauce, baked chicken, dinner roll, margarine, fruit cup, Perrier water, and after-dinner mint that made up the rest of the meal. All this food was digested, absorbed, and distributed to the tissues with surprisingly little disturbance in the concentration of glucose in the blood. Despite the transport of about 1,000 calories, including about 30,000 milligrams of glucose, the blood glucose concentration never even doubled from its pre-dinner level of 80–100 mg/dl.

At this point, although the absorption of glucose has finished, the drain of glucose from the bloodstream continues, as brain and other tissues continue to consume it. Because of this constant demand, there has to be a means of providing continuing glucose input into the bloodstream until the next meal is taken. Glycogen provides the means.

Glycogen acts as a reservoir of glucose molecules that the body calls upon once there is no more glucose coming in from the intestine. As glucose absorption ceases, insulin levels fall. The lack of insulin signals the liver to break glycogen down into individual glucose molecules, which flow into the bloodstream for use by the rest of the body. For several hours after absorption is complete, the liver continues to liberate glucose from its glycogen stores, thus providing the necessary glucose input and preventing hypoglycemia. Obviously if someone is unable to break glycogen down into glucose (which is the case in several inherited diseases[1]), hypoglycemia would occur unless food were taken very frequently.

Several hours after all food absorption has ceased (exactly how long depends on how big the last meal was and how much exercise has occurred), the liver starts to run out of glycogen. With no more glucose coming in from the intestines, and no more glycogen to convert to glucose, the body must call upon its third source of glucose input: gluconeogenesis.

Gluco means "glucose," of course; *neo* means "new"; *genesis* signifies "creation." *Gluconeogenesis,* then, is the creation of new glucose. The new glucose is created by the liver (and also the kidneys, especially during a prolonged fast), utilizing other basic

[1] **These conditions, known as "glycogen storage diseases," are explained in Chapter 8.**

foodstuffs suchs as lactic acid, amino acids from muscle, and glycerol from fat. Because the brain must have its constant supply of glucose, the body resorts to tearing its own tissues down—especially muscle—to keep the glucose flowing to the brain. Meanwhile, however, the tissues are switching their energy metabolism away from glucose and to the utilization of fat, in order to spare glucose for the brain.

In order to achieve gluconeogenesis, many body processes must work harmoniously. Amino acids must be liberated from muscle tissue and glycerol from fat. These ingredients must travel through the bloodstream to the liver. The cell machinery in the liver must be properly programmed to produce sugar for export rather than glycogen for storage. Hormones, especially glucagon and low levels of insulin, provide the coordinating signals so that the various tissues can each do their part. Unless all of these contributing steps are taken, hypoglycemia can result.

The statement that the liver manufactures glucose is a deceptively simple one. It's like driving past an automobile assembly plant and saying, "That's where Cadillacs are made." Even the further explanation that small simple parts come in one end of the factory and are carefully assembled so that complete cars emerge from the other end grossly understates the complexity of the operation. For the Cadillac plant to produce, countless factors must each contribute. Electricity must be generated at hydroelectric generating plants and travel to the plant over functioning power lines. Labor unions must agree to contracts and provide adequate skilled manpower. Subsidiary companies making batteries, tires, glass, paint, grease, steel, radios, heaters, air conditioners, and mufflers must all contribute on schedule. Transportation systems bringing parts and workers must operate reliably, and so forth. In fact, the more you know about the operation of a Cadillac factory, the more you realize how incredibly complex the whole process is. When you think that a breakdown can occur at any step along the way, it is amazing that complete cars ever come off the production line. Similarly, gluconeogenesis isn't as simple as it first sounds. Medical scientists are continually learning more details about the many individual steps involved. And the more one understands the whole process, the more amazing it is that it works. When one of the steps doesn't work, hypoglycemia can result.

The individual steps in gluconeogenesis are carried out by *enzymes*. Enzymes are specialized molecules that speed up chemical reactions. For example, one of the steps necessary to convert the amino acid named alanine into glucose is to remove a nitrogen atom from the alanine. Like other steps, this one is carried out by a specific enzyme. There are dozens of different enzymes involved in gluconeogenesis. Each one governs a specific step necessary for the production of glucose—just as each worker or robot in a Cadillac factory makes a specific contribution to the production of the car. When one of the enzymes is missing or defective, as in certain inherited conditions, glucose production may be blocked and the blood sugar may fall.

Not only gluconeogenesis, but all of the processes involved in the control of blood glucose depend on enzymes. As we have seen, digestive enzymes break down complex foods within the intestine into simple, absorbable molecules like glucose. Other enzymes, activated by insulin, govern glycogen production. Still others, inhibited by insulin and stimulated by glucagon, promote glycogen breakdown. It is largely through their ability to modify the activity of enzymes that drugs and hormones influence the processes that control blood sugar.

Before going on to a specific example of the function and malfunction of the processes we've discussed, let's review what we've covered so far:

1. Blood glucose levels depend on the balance between the *outflow* of glucose from blood into tissues, and the *input* of glucose from the intestine, from glycogen breakdown, and from gluconeogenesis.
2. Low blood sugar can result from accelerated glucose outflow, or from retarded input, or from both.

A high rate of glucose outflow, plus problems with all three sources of blood sugar input—absorption, glycogen breakdown, and gluconeogenesis—led to hypoglycemia in Sherry Tippler, a healthy middle-aged woman whose case is particularly instructive.

Early on a Saturday afternoon Mrs. Tippler decided to clean her refrigerator and freezer. She skipped lunch because she hadn't gotten up until ten that morning, when she had just her usual cup of coffee for breakfast.

She unplugged the refrigerator/freezer and carried its perishable contents over to a neighbor's home around 1:00 P.M. As the ice began to melt in her freezer, a large puddle formed on the floor, so Sherry decided she might as well scrub the floor. On her hands and knees she noticed that the walls and woodwork need scrubbing too, so she did them as well.

Her husband, Alex, had been watching football on TV in the living room. He went out for an early dinner at McDonald's, because there was nothing to eat in the house. Alex didn't bring any food home for Sherry, however, because he knew she was watching her weight.

The ice was slow to melt in the freezer, and it was not until 10:30 P.M. that the defrosting and cleaning job was done and the refrigerator plugged back in. By then it was too late to get the food back from the neighbors, who always went to bed early. Since there was nothing to munch on in the house, Sherry decided to keep working. The refrigerator done, it was time to wax the floor.

Sherry applied wax to the kitchen and breakfast-room floors. As the wax was drying she joined her husband in front of the TV to watch Johnny Carson. Aching and feeling tired, she had a few drinks of whiskey with her husband and then went back to the kitchen to polish the waxed floor. She hadn't been there more than 15 minutes when Alex called from the living room, "Sherry—come on in here! You've gotta see this comedy routine!" No answer came from the kitchen, so Mr. Tippler put down his drink and went to investigate. He found his wife slumped on the floor, pale, unconscious, and sweating profusely. He couldn't rouse her, so he frantically carried her to the car and drove to the nearby hospital emergency room.

The physician in the emergency room noted alcohol on Mrs. Tippler's breath and drew blood for measurement of alcohol level as well as a battery of chemistry tests, including measurement of the level of glucose. Then, as a matter of routine in such cases, he gave her a shot of thiamine, followed by an intravenous injection of glucose in water. Within thirty seconds Sherry regained consciousness. She was confused and combative for a couple of minutes, then gradually returned to normal.

When the laboratory technician phoned the results back to the emergency-room physician, it was obvious why Mrs. Tippler had been unconscious. Her plasma glucose level had fallen to 12 mg/dl!

The alcohol level was 185 mg/dl—enough to impair driving (the legal limit in most states is 100 mg/dl), but certainly not enough by itself to explain coma. Hypoglycemia was the cause of her unconsciousness.

Why did Mrs. Tippler's blood glucose fall so low? First of all, glucose outflow was rapid, because of her prolonged and vigorous exercise defrosting, scrubbing, waxing, and polishing. The rapid glucose outflow would not have caused hypoglycemia, however, unless glucose input were impaired. Let's look at each of the three possible sources of glucose input into Mrs. Tippler's bloodstream.

First, *absorption* of carbohydrates had completely ceased hours before. The teaspoon of sugar in her breakfast coffee at 10:00 A.M. had been completely absorbed before 11:00. Second, *glycogen* stores were depleted because it had been so long since she had replenished them by eating a good meal, and she had been using them up working hard all day. Ever since late afternoon, therefore, she had been relying solely on *gluconeogenesis* for input of glucose into her bloodstream. Then she did something that blocks gluconeogenesis: She drank alcohol.

Alcohol blocks the production of new glucose from amino acids and glycerol. As alcohol is burned up in the liver, it uses up a substance necessary for proper function of certain enzymes involved in gluconeogenesis. By thus stopping gluconeogenesis, alcohol produces hypoglycemia in anyone who has been fasting for a long time and has thereby depleted his or her stores of glycogen.

So, if you're going to have a few beers after a long hard day's work on an empty stomach, remember to eat the pretzels and peanuts. The starch from the pretzels will supply glucose for absorption. Without it, and with no glycogen available, an alcohol-induced block of gluconeogenesis will deprive you of your only source of blood glucose. Then, as the brain and other tissues continue their normal, necessary uptake of glucose, blood glucose levels will fall and symptoms will ensue.

As with Sherry Tippler, most cases of low blood sugar level result from a combination of several factors operating together to reduce the level of blood glucose. Hypoglycemia occurs when high rates of glucose *outflow* from the bloodstream combine with low glucose *input*.

Rapid glucose outflow occurs commonly in exercise and in pregnancy. Exercise, of course, increases the energy demands of muscle, and glucose flows more rapidly from blood into the muscles to supply this demand. Pregnancy is a special case of accelerated glucose outflow. The placenta, which transfers oxygen, glucose, and other nutrients from the mother to the fetus, acts as a glucose "sink." It continually drains glucose from the mother's circulation, thereby making the pregnant woman particularly susceptible to hypoglycemia. It also drains amino acids, such as alanine, needed for gluconeogenesis. The fetus appears to have first call on nutrients in the mother's bloodstream, so she must eat frequently to avoid hypoglycemia, especially in the first three months of pregnancy.

When one considers the balance between input and outflow, it is clear that anyone can avoid hypoglycemia by simply eating fast enough and often enough. It is between feedings that problems occur.

Three factors must be present to avoid between-meal hypoglycemia:

1. a healthy liver, where glycogen breakdown and gluconeogenesis can take place,
2. an adequate supply of basic building blocks, such as amino acids and glycerol, for the liver to utilize in manufacturing glucose, and
3. the proper mix of hormones to regulate the function of the liver and the availability of the building blocks.

The main hormones involved in the regulation of glucose metabolism are insulin, glucagon, growth hormone, cortisol, and adrenalin (also known as epinephrine). Excessive amounts of insulin, and deficiencies in the other hormones, can cause hypoglycemia. The remainder of this chapter will briefly explain the impact of each of these hormones on human glucose metabolism.

Insulin is the most important hormone influencing blood sugar. Too much produces hypoglycemia; too little produces high blood sugar.

Insulin lowers the blood glucose in several ways. First, it causes glucose coming in from the intestines to be captured and stored in the liver as glycogen, thus keeping it temporarily out of circulation. Second, it restrains glycogen breakdown. Third, it inhibits gluconeogenesis. Fourth, it facilitates the outflow of glucose from the blood into most tissues, including fat, muscle, and brain. All of these actions of insulin tend to lower blood glucose levels and to favor the storage and uptake of glucose in liver and tissues.

To use a basketball analogy, insulin may be said to put a "full court press" on your blood sugar; not only does it restrain glucose input at every point, it also speeds glucose outflow into body tissues.

Glucagon, like insulin, comes from the islets of Langerhans in the pancreas. Although some of its actions, such as the promotion of amino-acid uptake and protein production, resemble those of insulin, its effects on blood sugar are opposite to those of insulin. Therefore, glucagon, like growth hormone, cortisol, and adrenalin, is an "anti-insulin" or "counter-insulin" hormone.

Glucagon raises the blood sugar. It does this by promoting glycogen breakdown and gluconeogenesis, which increase the flow of glucose from the liver into the bloodstream. At the concentrations of glucagon normally present in man, the tendency of glucagon to raise blood sugar is not very strong, a fact that may explain why no definite cases of hypoglycemia caused solely by deficiency of glucagon have been discovered in humans. Glucagon, however, strongly influences blood sugar when given in large doses by injection. Such injections are used to treat some causes of hypoglycemia and produce glucagon levels much higher than normally occur in healthy persons.

Growth hormone comes from the pituitary gland, situated just beneath the brain as shown in Fig. 10. As its name implies, it promotes growth. Levels of growth hormone in the blood vary inversely to the concentration of glucose. A rise in blood sugar shuts off the secretion of growth hormone, and a fall in blood sugar stimulates the pituitary to secrete more growth hormone. For example, during a glucose tolerance test, growth hormone is normally shut off during the first hour, when blood sugar levels are rising, then is secreted vigorously when the blood sugar falls. The fall in blood sugar proceeds more rapidly if there is a deficiency of growth hormone, since growth hormone blocks the outflow of glucose into the tissues. It also appears to promote gluconeogenesis. In these ways growth hormone opposes the action of insulin.

Children who have a deficiency of growth hormone are prone to hypoglycemia. The fact that they are short for their age (be-

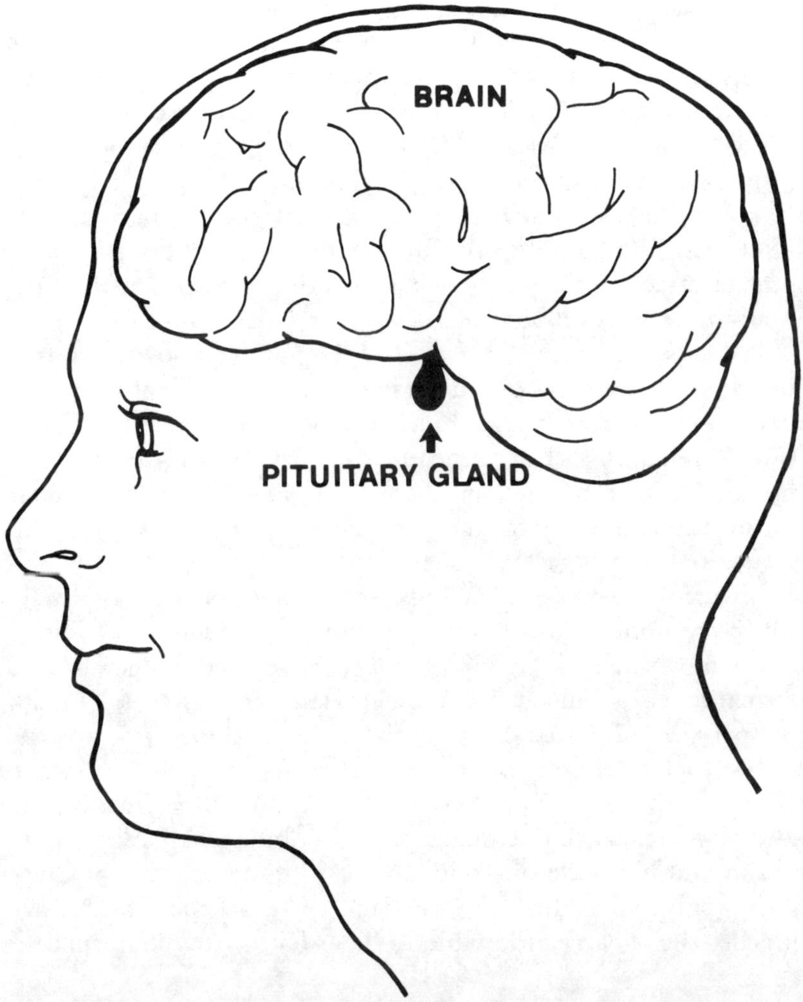

Fig. 10. The pituitary gland produces growth hormone and a hormone that stimulates the adrenal cortex to produce cortisol. Both of these hormones are important in glucose metabolism, and their lack may lead to hypoglycemia. The pituitary also produces several other important hormones that influence metabolism throughout the body.

cause of the lack of growth hormone) helps point toward the correct diagnosis. Adults with growth-hormone deficiency have less of a tendency toward hypoglycemia than children, but the reason for this difference is not known.

Cortisol comes from the outer shell, or cortex, of the adrenal glands, as shown earlier in Fig. 6. This was the hormone missing in the case of Enrique Engelhardt, recounted in Chapter 1. Cortisol raises the blood sugar by promoting gluconeogenesis and also by slowing glucose outflow into tissues. In addition, it has an indirect effect of enhancing the effects of glucagon and adrenalin in raising levels of blood sugar.

Adrenalin, otherwise known as epinephrine, also comes from the adrenal glands. As explained in Chapter 2, this is the hormone that causes adrenergic symptoms when the blood glucose falls too low. Adrenalin blocks the secretion of insulin from the pancreas, thus affecting both input and outflow of glucose. It also stimulates the breakdown of glycogen into glucose, further flooding the circulation with sugar.

Despite these powerful actions, adrenalin does not play a major role in the minute-to-minute regulation of blood glucose. Rather, it is a mechanism kept in reserve to raise blood sugar back to normal levels should it become necessary. In this sense it is like the spare can of gasoline kept in the trunk of your car: It does not supply fuel to the engine on a daily basis but gets you out of trouble if the main tank runs dry. Because adrenalin does not normally regulate blood sugar on a continuing basis, lack of adrenalin and blockade of its action by drugs are not major causes of hypoglycemia. Instead, the lack or blockade of adrenalin impedes the *recovery* of low blood sugar levels back to normal.

SUMMARY

To summarize the main points of this chapter:

1. The level of blood glucose is a balance between input and outflow.
2. Hypoglycemia results when glucose input falls relative to outflow.
3. Glucose constantly flows out of the bloodstream to the brain and other tissues. Insulin, exercise, and pregnancy increase the rate of glucose outflow.

4. Absorption of glucose from the intestines, liberation of glucose from glycogen, and manufacture of new glucose all contribute to input.
5. In order to maintain glucose input and normal glucose levels in the blood after the absorption of food has ceased, three factors are essential:
   a. a healthy liver,
   b. adequate supplies of building blocks (such as amino acids) in the bloodstream for the manufacture of glucose in the liver, and
   c. proper amounts of hormones to integrate and regulate the processes of glucose metabolism.

   The lack of any of these factors leads to hypoglycemia in the fasting state.
6. Alcohol stops the liver from manufacturing new glucose, and can therefore cause hypoglycemia.

In the next two chapters we shall examine other causes of low blood sugar.

7

What Causes Hypoglycemia in Adults?

Hypoglycemia doesn't "just happen." If your blood sugar is abnormally low, there's a reason for it.

The processes that govern glucose input and outflow were reviewed in the last chapter. They are complex. And as in many complex systems, Murphy's Law reigns supreme.

Murphy's Law holds that anything that *can* go wrong *will* go wrong. The law applies to aviation (sooner or later some mechanic will install a propeller backward, etc.), military operations, communications, and many other enterprises with interdependent parts. It applies equally well to human metabolism. Sooner or later, each of the steps in the regulation of blood glucose will go wrong. In some cases a built-in protective mechanism may compensate for the error. In other cases, too high or too low a level of glucose will result. If the blood sugar is consistently too high, we call the resulting syndrome diabetes mellitus. If the blood sugar is too low, *hypoglycemia* exists. In either case, we must seek the underlying cause so we can take appropriate corrective action.

Table 2 lists many of the causes of hypoglycemia. It groups these causes into two categories depending on whether the action speeds up glucose outflow or interferes with glucose input. The rest of this chapter follows the outline of Table 2, so if you get sidetracked in the details, you can get back on track by referring to the table.

Table 2

CAUSES OF HYPOGLYCEMIA CHARACTERISTICALLY OCCURRING IN ADULTS

I. *ACCELERATED GLUCOSE OUTFLOW*
   A. EXERCISE
   B. PREGNANCY, ESPECIALLY FIRST THREE MONTHS
   C. INSULIN AND RELATED CAUSES
   D. SEVERE, WIDESPREAD INFECTION

II. *IMPAIRED GLUCOSE INPUT*
   A. SUBSTANCES THAT LOWER BLOOD SUGAR
      1. *INSULIN*
         a) Externally Administered Insulin
         b) Internally Secreted Insulin
            (1) Tumors
            (2) Reactive hypoglycemia
               (a) Reactive hypoglycemia of known cause
                  i) previous ulcer surgery
                  ii) oral glucose tolerance tests and similar meals
                  iii) sugar and alcohol
               (b) Reactive hypoglycemia of unknown cause ("idiopathic")
      2. *DRUGS THAT WORK THROUGH INSULIN*
      3. *OTHER DRUGS*
      4. *UNRIPE ACKEE FRUIT*
      5. *ALCOHOL*
      6. *INTERNALLY PRODUCED SUBSTANCES THAT ACT LIKE INSULIN*
         a) Tumors
         b) Antibodies to Insulin Receptors
         c) Antibodies to Insulin
   B. LACK OF SUBSTANCES THAT RAISE BLOOD SUGAR
      1. *ADRENAL-GLAND FAILURE*
      2. *PITUITARY-GLAND FAILURE*
      3. *GLUCAGON DEFICIENCY*
   C. PROLONGED, SEVERE STARVATION
   D. LIVER FAILURE
   E. KIDNEY FAILURE
   F. SEVERE CONGESTIVE HEART FAILURE
   G. SEVERE, WIDESPREAD INFECTION

Although we shall discuss the causes of hypoglycemia one at a time, in most actual instances of hypoglycemia a combination of several causes works together. A glance at Table 2 reveals that most causes of hypoglycemia arise from a deficiency of glucose input. Less frequently, hypoglycemia arises primarily from excessive glucose outflow.

I. ACCELERATED GLUCOSE OUTFLOW

A. EXERCISE

Actively contracting muscles extract glucose from the bloodstream and burn it up as fuel. This drains glucose from the circulation, and often triggers an episode of low blood sugar in someone who already has a tendency toward hypoglycemia. Most normal people compensate for exercise by speeding up glucose production and by switching over to alternative energy sources such as fat. Therefore, exercise does not normally cause hypoglycemia. But when a problem exists with glucose production or fat metabolism, exercise often brings on an attack. This is what happened to Mrs. Tippler, as recounted in the last chapter. The exercise of all that housework caused glucose to flow out of her bloodstream, and alcohol then blocked the production of new glucose. The combination of increased glucose outflow and blocked input produced hypoglycemia.

Severe and prolonged exercise can lower the blood sugar into the 20s in some normal people, but no hypoglycemic symptoms occur because blood is pumping rapidly (remember that glucose delivery to the brain is the product of *both* blood glucose concentration and the rate of blood flow), and because the body's metabolism makes use of other fuels that are abundant during exercise. However, if the marathon runner were to celebrate his victory with a bottle of champagne immediately after the race, the alcohol would block glucose input from the liver, and blood sugar would fall still further.

B. PREGNANCY, ESPECIALLY FIRST THREE MONTHS

Many women experience hypoglycemia for the first time in early pregnancy and find themselves heading for the refrigerator at 3:00 A.M. The fetus takes sugar, as well as amino acids needed for gluconeogenesis, from the mother's bloodstream. As a consequence, hypoglycemia commonly occurs in the first three months of pregnancy. At this early stage of pregnancy, food intake is often curtailed by nausea. Moreover, the hormones of pregnancy (which raise blood sugar) are not so abundant then as they will be later on.

Women with diabetes mellitus who take insulin to bring their blood glucose down to normal are especially liable to drop their blood sugar too low in early pregnancy. The case of Margo illustrates this common problem.

Margo, who had been diabetic since age 12, took injections of insulin twice each day. She watched her diet carefully, exercised regularly every day, and had frequent blood tests to check the level of her blood sugar. She was doing a beautiful job of keeping her levels of blood glucose down to normal or only a little above normal. She rarely had symptoms of too low a blood sugar from overtreatment.

Two years after she married Bob, Margo became pregnant. Since her menstrual periods were often irregular, coming anywhere from four to eight weeks apart, Margo didn't suspect she was pregnant until she woke up with intense nausea several days in a row. By then she had been pregnant almost a month. When she called her friend's gynecologist, the receptionist informed her that the first opening for an appointment was three weeks away.

The week before she was due at the doctor's office, Margo had a bad heachache. It started one morning when she awoke. She felt exhausted. Bob told her she had slept restlessly during the night and had seemed to be having a bad dream. As she thought back, she remembered a nightmare and supposed that was why she felt so tired.

Neither Bob nor Margo gave these symptoms any more thought that day. The next night, however, Bob was awakened around 4:00 A.M. by the bed shaking. As he awoke, he realized Margo was shaking. Her eyes were rolled back, her skin was moist, and she was unconscious. Bob suspected hypoglycemia and ran to the kitchen to get some Coca-Cola with added sugar to pour into her mouth. He couldn't get her to swallow any of it, so he called an ambulance.

When the paramedics arrived, Bob told them Margo was diabetic and took insulin injections. The paramedics recognized this as a probable case of hypoglycemia and promptly inserted a needle into a vein in Margo's arm. They drew a tube full of blood for later laboratory analysis, and gave her glucose intravenously. The shaking stopped and Margo woke up gradually over the next three minutes. They took her to a hospital emergency room, where analysis of the blood drawn from her arm showed a glucose level of 18 mg/dl. She had indeed been hypoglycemic.

Why had hypoglycemia developed without any change in Margo's exercise or insulin dosage? The answer was in her uterus: The baby was drawing glucose out of Margo's blood glucose. The insulin she was taking prevented her liver from making additional glucose to compensate for the drain of glucose to the fetus.

Margo's doctor admitted her to the hospital in order to make the necessary adjustments in her diet and insulin dosage. He increased the amount of food she ate for a bedtime snack and reduced the dose of her evening shot of insulin. With less insulin and more food, Margo's blood sugar remained above hypoglycemic levels.

The nightmares and the morning headaches stopped. They were probably symptoms of Margo's low blood sugar prior to the seizure that finally brought her to medical attention. Since the cause of her seizure had been hypoglycemia, prevention of hypoglycemia was all that was needed to avoid further seizures.

Margo's case illustrates the fact that more than one cause usually contributes to any particular instance of low blood sugar. In Margo's case it was a combination of increased glucose outflow (caused by pregnancy and insulin) and of decreased input (caused by insulin).

C. INSULIN AND RELATED CAUSES

Insulin (and, indirectly, other drugs that work through the body's own insulin) speeds the flow of glucose out of the bloodstream and into body tissues. Insulin is the most powerful determinant of the rate at which glucose leaves the bloodstream. Since insulin also slows the input of glucose into the circulation, it is discussed further in the next major section of this chapter.

D. SEVERE, WIDESPREAD INFECTION

Especially in babies, low blood sugar sometimes accompanies overwhelming infection spread by the bloodstream throughout the body. Hypoglycemia resulting from widespread infection is not well understood, but some evidence indicates that glucose flows from the bloodstream at an increased rate, perhaps into muscle, into the white blood cells fighting the infection, or into the infecting bacteria themselves. In some infections, such as certain severe cases of malaria, the bloodstream contains abnormally high levels of insulin.

II. IMPAIRED GLUCOSE INPUT

A. SUBSTANCES THAT LOWER BLOOD SUGAR

1. *INSULIN*

Insulin reduces blood sugar levels in four ways. First, insulin diverts glucose into the liver, where it is stored as animal starch (glycogen). Second, insulin inhibits the breakdown of glycogen into glucose. Third, insulin slows the production of new glucose (gluconeogenesis). These three actions of insulin all reduce the input of glucose into the bloodstream. Fourth, insulin accelerates the delivery of glucose from the bloodstream into body tissues. These four separate effects of insulin all combine to produce a powerful lowering of blood glucose levels. Consequently, excessive amounts of insulin are a major cause of hypoglycemia.

a) Externally Administered Insulin

Recent newspaper stories tell of a doctor accused of trying to murder his wife by injecting her with insulin. The prosecution wanted to prove that he had first drugged her with sedatives and then injected her with insulin to lower her blood sugar. The intent, they claimed, was to lower her blood sugar enough to produce severe brain damage and death. Whether true or not, this plot would certainly not qualify as a "perfect crime."

Insulin has serious shortcomings as a murder weapon. Chemical tests can distinguish insulin administered by injection from insulin secreted by one's own pancreas. Moreover, death may not ensue even if coma and brain damage occur. The vital breathing center of the brain resists damage by hypoglycemia more than many other areas of the brain.

Occasionally a patient with psychological problems intentionally inflicts hypoglycemia on himself. For one reason or another, certain unhappy individuals make themselves sick on purpose and then conceal the cause from their doctor. Whether it be for insurance money or for the care and sympathy that illness begets, some people take insulin on the sly. One such instance involved a 36-

year-old woman who had worked previously in a doctor's office. I shall call her L.G.

Late one Friday afternoon, L.G. arrived by ambulance at the hospital emergency room in apparent coma. Blood drawn for glucose measurement gave a reading of 26 mg/dl, definitely low. She "came to" after an intravenous injection of glucose. The intern listened to her complicated tale, which included fainting spells, episodes of hunger, headache, sweating, shakiness, and confusion. She omitted from her story the fact that she had previously been in a mental hospital. The intern didn't suspect any psychiatric problems, because her personality seemed perfectly normal. She was pleasant and rational and cooperative.

The intern admitted L.G. to a hospital ward with 16 beds in the same room and a nursing station in the center. Such a setting favored close and constant observation.

During the first 36 hours of hospitalization L.G. remained well. Visitors came and went. She ate normally and walked with nurses in the hallway. The intern hoped that one of her spells would occur while he or the nurses observed her, so they could measure her blood sugar and record her blood pressure, heartbeat, and any seizure activity.

Sunday morning as the nurses made their usual 6:00 A.M. rounds, they found L.G. in bed, unconscious and sweating profusely. Her heart rate was a rapid 140 beats per minute. Their efforts to rouse her failed, so they put in an emergency call for the intern. His examination confirmed her comatose condition, but showed no other problems besides the rapid heartbeat and sweating that are typical of severe hypoglycemia. He drew enough blood for measurement of both insulin and glucose. Then he injected into her vein a large amount of glucose, and watched her wake up.

She recovered consciousness, confused at first but then clear and calm. She couldn't recall anything about what had led up to the episode except that she'd had some unpleasant dreams that night. The lab reported her blood sugar level as 16 mg/dl. It would be several days before the insulin measurement became available.

Later that day a glucose tolerance test was done, with normal results. Several days passed and no further episodes occurred, even though at one point she was kept fasting for 48 hours. At the end of the 48-hour fast, during which she was allowed to take nothing by mouth except water, her blood sugar was a very normal 66 mg/dl.

The laboratory reported her insulin level, drawn Sunday morning with a simultaneous glucose level of 16 mg/dl, as being abnormally high. When blood glucose levels are low, insulin levels should be low also, unless the patient is taking insulin or some other drug that stimulates insulin secretion, or has a tumor of the pancreas that produces too much insulin. With this latter possibility in mind, the doctor sent L.G. to the X-ray department for special X-rays of her pancreas. No tumor was seen on the X-rays.

While L.G. was in the X-ray department, the intern and nurses searched her bed and clothes and bedside table for evidence of insulin or some other drug that she might be taking to lower her blood sugar. The search turned up nothing. The radiologist, however, discovered the clue that eventually solved the puzzle: Some abnormal shadows showed up on one of the X-rays of the abdomen. The X-ray technician had neglected to place the usual lead shield over the lower abdomen during one of the X-ray films, and in the area of the pelvis the X-ray revealed the needle of a syringe, and the metal cap of a bottle that later turned out to contain insulin. L.G. had been concealing them in her vagina! She had surreptitiously injected herself with insulin, and, since it takes several minutes for the insulin to begin to take effect, she'd had plenty of time to hide the evidence in her vagina before lapsing into coma.

After consulting a psychiatrist, the intern gently confronted L.G. with the evidence, and she admitted what she had been doing. This led to an outpouring of the psychological pressures she had been feeling. She resumed psychotherapy, which turned out to be the appropriate treatment for this case of hypoglycemia.

L.G.'s disease was not hypoglycemia. Low blood sugar was simply one manifestation of her psychological problems. Proper treatment depended on identifying her specific emotional and psychological problems, so that these could be addressed in a helpful way.

b) Internally Secreted Insulin

(1) Tumors

Specialized nests of cells within the pancreas known as the "islets of Langerhans" (named after their discoverer) manufacture insulin. These insulin-producing "islet cells," like most cells in the body, occasionally grow and operate in an uncontrolled manner—that is to say, they form tumors. When such tumors spread throughout the body, invading and destroying other tissues, they are called "malignant" tumors, or cancer. Other tumors are "benign," in the sense that they do not spread and destroy other tissues. Whether benign or malignant, tumors of the islet cells make their presence known by the hormones they secrete. Islet-cell tumors that secrete insulin are known as "insulinomas." They are an important, though unusual, cause of hypoglycemia.

Fortunately, effective treatment exists for insulinoma. The case of Juan Dominguez illustrates some of the benefits of accurate diagnosis of this cause of hypoglycemia.

Juan had a good work record but a history of intermittent psychiatric problems. He was prone to spells of withdrawal in which he would remain sullen and silent for hours or even days at a time. These spells led to his admission to the psychiatric ward of a large county hospital.

The psychiatrist who took care of him found he was often conversant and willing to discuss his feelings and past experiences. At other times, however, he seemed totally withdrawn.

The psychiatrist diagnosed Juan as a "catatonic schizophrenic." Medications were tried but didn't help much. In his normal periods, Juan told the psychiatrist of his early childhood and home situation. He had been a battered and abused child and still found it difficult to express or accept affection. This history reinforced the psychiatrist's impression that Juan's behavior was rooted in deep psychological problems.

Because drugs didn't help much, Juan eventually left the hospital on no medications at all. His outpatient treatment consisted of occasional counseling sessions with a therapist.

At work almost a year later, Juan went into a severe bout of withdrawal. It frightened his co-workers, who described his state as being like a "zombie"—his eyes were open yet he seemed paralyzed and either unconscious or very far away mentally. They brought him to a nearby community hospital while he was still in this trance, and he was admitted to the psychiatric ward with a diagnosis of "catatonia." This time the psychiatrist caring for Juan ordered a routine series of blood tests to be drawn the next morning before breakfast.

The blood test revealed a fasting plasma glucose level of 21 mg/dl! The psychiatrist promptly consulted an endocrinologist, who eventually diagnosed an insulin-secreting tumor. Until the operation, however, the doctors didn't know whether Juan's insulinoma was benign or malignant.

When the surgeon opened Juan's abdomen he found a lump in the pancreas about the size of a small acorn. He found no other lumps and no sign that the tumor had spread to the liver. The surgeon removed the portion of the pancreas that contained the lump. It turned out to be a benign insulinoma, and Juan was cured of his disease by its removal. He had no more spells of withdrawal or catatonia. His blood sugar remained normal, and he had no further psychiatric problems.

Unlike the case of L.G., who needed psychotherapy to get at the root of her hypoglycemia, Juan did not need psychotherapy. He needed an operation on his pancreas. Definition of the specific cause of the hypoglycemia allowed his doctors to provide specific and appropriate treatment.

(2) Reactive hypoglycemia

"Reactive" hypoglycemia means low blood sugar *after eating*. This is the most misunderstood and overdiagnosed type of hypoglycemia. Most actual cases of reactive hypoglycemia have a definite, identifiable cause. Reactive hypoglycemia of *unknown* cause, however, remains an area of rampant *mis*diagnosis and raging controversy.

(a) Reactive hypoglycemia of known cause

Almost any cause of hypoglycemia can lower blood glucose after meals and thus show a "reactive" pattern. A few causes of hypoglycemia, however, operate *only* after food intake. These are (i) rapid stomach emptying due to previous surgery for ulcers, (ii) a large dose of refined, readily absorbed carbohydrate taken on an empty stomach, and (iii) simultaneous intake of sugar and alcohol. Before examining them individually, let's review what they have in common.

In these three types of reactive hypoglycemia, the pancreas secretes large quantities of insulin while the meal is being absorbed. Then, food absorption stops fairly abruptly. With little or no continuing absorption of glucose, the high insulin levels drive the blood sugar down and a brief period of "overshoot" occurs as hypoglycemic levels are reached. Insulin levels then drop, and anti-insulin hormones act, bringing the blood sugar back up to normal.

You can reproduce this same pattern of response with intravenous glucose. If you take someone who hasn't eaten for several hours and experimentally administer large amounts of sugar by vein for a prolonged period, that person's blood glucose level will rise. The high blood glucose level will stimulate the person's pancreas to secrete insulin, and blood insulin levels will rise. Then, if you suddenly stop the infusion of glucose, the blood sugar will plummet because there is no incoming glucose to oppose the effects of all that insulin. The blood sugar will keep nosediving until *low* blood sugar signals the pancreas to turn off insulin. Then, probably with some help from anti-insulin hormones, the blood sugar will come back up to normal. If no additional cause of hypoglycemia is present, the blood sugar will return to normal within 10 to 25 minutes. This is also true of the known causes of purely reactive hypoglycemia: The periods of low blood sugar last only about 20 minutes or less. If the blood sugar stays low for longer than that, additional causes of hypoglycemia are at work.

i) previous ulcer surgery

"Alimentary hypoglycemia" describes low blood sugar in people who have had stomach surgery for ulcers. Several types of operations to relieve ulcers cause the stomach to empty its contents rapidly into the small intestine. Instead of acting as a holding tank, the surgically altered stomach discharges its contents quickly downstream into the intestine, which absorbs glucose rapidly. This flood of sugar coming into the bloodstream provokes the pancreas to put out lots of insulin. Additionally, the intestine releases exaggerated amounts of insulin-boosting hormones that further stimulate the pancreas. The result is a rapid rise in insulin levels followed by a rapid fall in blood sugar because of the insulin. Sometimes the blood sugar falls to hypoglycemic levels, especially if the carbohydrate was taken in the form of refined simple sugars, which are more quickly absorbed than complex starches with vegetable fiber. The abrupt cessation of sugar absorption, at a time when insulin levels are high, sets the stage for a downward "overshoot" of the level of blood sugar. The case of Lars Jensen typifies this problem of alimentary hypoglycemia.

About 10:00 A.M. on a Saturday morning, Mr. Jensen felt faint, weak, and clammy, and had a rapid heartbeat. He had eaten pancakes with syrup and jam, skim milk, and a glass of orange juice at about 8:30 A.M. Then he took his children to the park and was playing catch when the symptoms began. He felt so sick that he stopped playing with the children and sat down to rest for about 20 minutes. Similar episodes had occurred occasionally over the previous two years, especially on weekends, when he was more likely to eat a very sugary breakfast.

His past medical history included surgery for ulcers almost four years earlier. The surgeon had removed part of his stomach, enlarged the exit pathway from the stomach to the small intestine, and severed the nerve that normally retards stomach emptying.

Lars's story sounded to me like alimentary hypoglycemia. We decided to find out. Fortunately for Mr. Jensen we knew the facts discussed in Chapter 5 of this book, so he didn't have to endure the misery of a glucose tolerance test.

On the next Saturday, Lars again ate a breakfast rich in refined carbohydrates at 8:30 A.M. This time, instead of going to the park, he drove to my office, where we drew blood for sugar measurement at 10:00 A.M., 10:15 A.M., and again at 10:25 when he started to sweat and tremble and to feel very weak. The glucose level was 99 mg/dl at 10:00 A.M., 60 mg/dl at 10:15, and 37 mg/dl at 10:25. He drank a glass of orange juice and ate some cookies at 10:26, and by 10:32 he was looking and feeling better. A repeat blood sugar at that time was 64 mg/dl. His symptoms seemed to correspond to his blood glucose levels, drawn after his usual food intake, and I made a tentative diagnosis of alimentary hypoglycemia. His symptoms disappeared when he changed his diet pattern. By avoiding large amounts of refined sugar, and eating smaller and more balanced meals with higher fat, protein, and fiber content, he avoided further recurrence of his alarming experience in the park.

Remember, however, that not everyone with similar symptoms and a history of stomach surgery has hypoglycemia. The symptoms are not unique to low blood sugar, so you *must* make measurements. Rapid stomach emptying can cause intestinal cramping, sweating, and a feeling of faintness in what is known as "dumping syndrome" without any abnormal drop in the blood sugar. To make the diagnosis of alimentary hypoglycemia, a demonstrably low level of blood sugar must occur after the patient's usual dietary intake. An oral glucose tolerance test usually causes marked hypoglycemia in such a person, but since it causes hypoglycemia so often in normal people as well, its use confuses rather than clarifies the problem.

Many doctors believe that cases similar to this occur even in the absence of previous stomach surgery. The leading theory is that rapid stomach emptying (for some other reason, such as an overactive thyroid gland that speeds up many body processes) produces the same sequence of rapid absorption, insulin release, and downward overshoot of the blood sugar. Unfortunately, very few cases have been documented to have a definitely low level of blood sugar measured after the patient's normal meals. Instead, the diagnosis has relied on the glucose tolerance test, which is treacherously unreliable, and on symptoms not specific to hypoglycemia.[1] Thus, if alimentary hypoglycemia in the absence of gastrointestinal surgery exists at all, it must be exceedingly rare.

Based on the theory that rapid stomach emptying is the cause of some cases of "reactive hypoglycemia," physicians have prescribed pills, such as propantheline, that slow the emptying of the stomach.[1,2] That some patients experience a lessening of their symptoms does not prove that their blood sugar was abnormally low in the first place. Published results contain no carefully designed scientific studies using such drugs along with placebos to control for the effects of psychological suggestion. Consequently, in the absence of prior stomach surgery, the diagnosis of reactive hypoglycemia due to rapid stomach emptying remains controversial.

ii) oral glucose tolerance tests and similar meals

The oral glucose tolerance test is a frequent, though unpredictable, *cause* of hypoglycemia. Like the man we met in Chapter 5 who ate his waffles in a cereal bowl, some people frequently insult their systems with food resembling a glucose tolerance test. Insulin levels rise not only because the sugar stimulates the pancreas, but also because the small intestine releases insulin-boosting hormones. The larger the blast of carbohydrate calories hitting the intestine, the greater the output of these hormones. Consequently, a large dose of readily absorbed carbohydrate produces the full effect. A small dose of sugar, such as a couple of Life-Savers, doesn't.

[1] **M. A. Permutt et al., *New England Journal of Medicine* 288 (1973), 1206.**
[2] **M. A. Permutt, D. Keller, and J. Santiago, *Diabetes* 26 (1977), 121.**

Fat or protein in the meal slow the evacuation of the stomach, thus prolonging the period of absorption and reducing the likelihood of hypoglycemia. Continuing absorption of glucose then prevents the blood sugar level from falling as fast and as far. Intake of vegetable fiber such as bran and cellulose also slows the absorption of carbohydrate. The slower the absorption, the less the rise in levels of blood sugar and insulin, and the less likely it is that a downward rebound will occur. You can thus see how normally balanced meals, and the inclusion of complex starches rather than simple sugars, prevent this type of reactive hypoglycemia. By providing sustained absorption of glucose, continued nibbling will also prevent the blood sugar from falling.

iii) sugar and alcohol

We have seen in the case of Mrs. Tippler how alcohol blocks gluconeogenesis and causes *fasting* hypoglycemia. Alcohol has still other actions that contribute to the development of *reactive* hypoglycemia. Alcohol impairs the secretion of growth hormone from the pituitary gland and promotes the secretion of insulin from the pancreas. Both these actions reduce blood sugar. Consequently, when alcohol is present, intake of an amount of sugar considerably less than a glucose tolerance test can produce reactive hypoglycemia. This phenomenon has been called "gin and tonic" hypoglycemia, since the gin supplies the alcohol and the tonic supplies the sugar. The same problem can occur with any similar combination. Whiskey and ginger ale, rum and Coca-Cola, sweet wine, and beer with bar nibbles that are composed of quickly absorbable carbohydrate can all produce hypoglycemia when taken on an empty stomach. Dr. Vincent Marks, a foremost researcher on the subject of alcohol-induced hypoglycemia, points out that these facts throw "grave doubt on the wisdom of the age-old practice of using large amounts of sweetened coffee or tea to hasten 'sobering-up,' e.g. in preparation for a long drive home after a convivial evening during which alcohol, but little solid food, has been consumed."[3] He also observes that sweeteners that do not provoke insulin secretion, such as saccharin and fructose, do not lead to reactive hypoglycemia when combined with alcohol.

[3] **V. Marks, "Alchohol-induced hypoglycemia," in V. Marks and F. C. Rose, *Hypoglycemia*, 2nd ed. (Oxford: Blackwell Scientific Publications, 1981), 394.**

(b) Reactive hypoglycemia of unknown cause ("idiopathic")

The word "idiopathic" means "we don't know the cause." It is one of several terms used by the medical profession to disguise ignorance by dressing it up with a title. "Idiopathic reactive hypoglycemia" means "low blood sugar of unknown cause after meals."

Idiopathic reactive hypoglycemia is like a mystery guest at a masquerade ball. Glimpsed by everyone, comprehended by no one, he appears to be everywhere. When at last unmasked by scientific scrutiny, he usually proves to be an impostor.

Idiopathic reactive hypoglycemia doubtless does exist. Excluding insulinoma, stomach surgery, abnormal diet, alcohol, hereditary fructose intolerance, and all the other *known* causes of reactive hypoglycemia, there are no doubt some people who have low blood sugar after meals. Medical science has surely not discovered all the causes of reactive hypoglycemia. On the other hand, well-proved cases of idiopathic reactive hypoglycemia (diagnosed by definitely low levels of blood sugars measured after normal meals, and not just during glucose tolerance tests) are *few and far between*.

The great popular misconception is that idiopathic reactive hypoglycemia is a common condition. The treatment usually prescribed is a diet appropriate for victims of alimentary hypoglycemia due to previous stomach surgery: low-carbohydrate, high-protein, frequent feedings. Sometimes other treatments, such as an inactive extract of animal adrenal glands, vitamins, and trace mineral supplements, substitute for or join the diet. In the great majority of cases, neither the diagnosis nor the treatment is well founded. Most people labeled with the diagnosis have not been shown to have abnormally low blood glucose levels during their day-to-day symptoms. If they had, a scientific evaluation to find the known causes of hypoglycemia would have been in order. Instead, the usual diagnosis rests merely on symptoms or glucose tolerance tests. Stella Sharp, in Chapter 5, is a case in point.

Most people with symptoms after eating that resemble those of hypoglycemia do not, in fact, have low blood sugar. When scientifically tested, their glucose metabolism usually turns out to be normal. When it is abnormal, a specific cause can usually be identified. An excellent textbook for doctors on hypoglycemia, written by experts at the Mayo Clinic, summarized "idiopathic reactive hypoglycemia" as follows:

> Hypoglycemia as a nondisease has reached epidemic proportions (Yager and Young 1974). This can be traced to its popularization by magazine articles, health food publications, and self-styled nutritionists as the basis for many of humankind's ailments. There is a desire among many people to have a socially acceptable medical disorder that is easily and painlessly treated. Individuals with the false diagnosis of hypoglycemia also frequently suffer from food non-allergies and non-hypovitaminosis.[4]

To lay all the blame for overdiagnosis of idiopathic reactive hypoglycemia on patients and the popular media, however, is unfair. The medical profession must bear some of the responsibility for not recognizing sooner the illogic and unreliability of glucose tolerance testing as a means of diagnosing hypoglycemia. Part of the failure no doubt originates in the pressures felt by physicians to come up with a specific diagnosis.

When confronted with complaints of unknown cause, some doctors have told patients their problems were apparently due to hypoglycemia. In certain instances this has provided comfort to both patient and physician by relieving fears that the doctor didn't know what was going on and therefore couldn't help cure the patient. If patient or physician desired substantiation of low blood sugar, the glucose tolerance test was easily available for misuse and misdiagnosis, providing "proof" of the reactive hypoglycemia.

The therapies for idiopathic reactive hypoglycemia have in many cases not hurt the patient. Indeed, many patients misdiagnosed as having reactive hypoglycemia have felt better on the prescribed treatment. This may have been a direct effect of the treatment, or an indirect "placebo" benefit. In neither case, however, does it prove that the patient really had low blood sugar in the first place (except perhaps during the glucose tolerance test, which causes hypoglycemia in healthy normal people).

I have no objection to people feeling better on treatment. I do object, however, to a delusion that retards medical progress and wastes patients' time and money in pursuit of a cure for a disease they do not have.

[4] M. J. Hogan and F. J. Service, "Reactive Hypoglycemias" in F. J. Service, ed., *Hypoglycemic Disorders; Pathogenesis, Diagnosis and Treatment* (Boston: G. K. Hall Medical Publishers, 1983), 169.

Some doctors will counter defensively that their use of the diagnosis of reactive hypoglycemia falls into "the art rather than the science of medicine." This no doubt applies to much of what we do today as doctors, including the bedside manner. In the last century the "art of medicine" made use of leeches to bleed people as a cure for disease. Many of those people felt much better after being bled. It's a sobering thought that we in this new century send patients for six-hour bleeding sessions at clinical laboratories where white-clad leeches sweeten the experience with an initial bottle of glucose syrup.

Some prominent authors will disagree with my statement that idiopathic reactive hypoglycemia is uncommon.[5] These authors, however, define their patients as having hypoglycemia according to the results of glucose tolerance testing. For the reasons reviewed in Chapters 4 and 5, the glucose tolerance test is not a rational way to diagnose reactive hypoglycemia. It *is* a way to *produce* temporary hypoglycemia, but not a good way to elucidate the nature of patients' daily symptoms. Equally prominent authors discourage the use of the OGTT as a means of diagnosing hypoglycemia, and correctly insist on the finding of low blood glucose during everyday symptoms, with relief of symptoms as the blood sugar is raised.[6–8]

Lacking evidence of low blood sugar during spontaneously occuring symptoms, some popularizers of idiopathic reactive hypoglycemia have latched onto this notion: "The blood sugar need not be low so long as it is *falling* rapidly." This idea that a *rapid descent of the blood sugar* within the normal range constitutes hypoglycemia is *false*. In the first place, hypoglycemia *means* low blood sugar, not a falling blood sugar. In the second place, no one has ever shown that the rate of fall of the blood glucose within the normal range during ordinary living gives rise to spontaneous symptoms. We are really talking here about a hypothetical new

[5] P. S. Rotwein, S. J. Giddings, and M. A. Permutt, "Diagnosis and Management of Hypoglycemic Disorders in Adults," in M. P. Cohen and P. P. Foa, eds., *Special Topics in Endocrinology and Metabolism*, vol. 3 (New York: Alan R. Liss, Inc., 1982), 87.

[6] F. J. Service, "Clinical Presentation and Laboratory Evaluation of Hypoglycemic Disorders in Adults," in F. J. Service, ed., *Hypoglycemic Disorders; Pathogenesis, Diagnosis and Treatment* (Boston: G. K. Hall Medical Publishers, 1983), 74.

[7] V. Marks, "The Investigation of Hypoglycemia," in V. Marks and F. C. Rose, eds., *Hypoglycemia*, 2nd ed. (Oxford: Blackwell Scientific Publications, 1981), 443.

[8] D. D. Johnson et al., *Journal of the American Medical Association* 243 (1980), 1151.

disease—one that has *never been shown to exist,* except as an unusual feature of chronic, severe diabetes mellitus (high blood sugar).[9] If it were found to exist, it might be called "adrenergic discomfort arising from rapidly falling levels of blood glucose," not hypoglycemia.

Many people do have adrenergic symptoms with normal blood glucose levels. It has never been demonstrated, however, that any of these people experience these symptoms only when their blood glucose is descending at a certain rate, and not when it is falling more slowly. Thus, there is no rate of glucose decline within the normal range, in mg/dl per minute, that defines whether or not someone will develop adrenergic symptoms. The question has been studied in detail with oral and intravenous glucose administration as well as insulin to produce falling levels of blood sugar. In those tests, some scientists have found that adrenalin secretion increased only after the blood sugar reached hypoglycemic levels,[10] whereas others reported that adrenalin increased while the blood sugar was falling within or above the normal range.[11,12] The rate of fall, however, did not correlate with the amount of adrenalin released. Instead, what determined the amount of adrenalin released was how low the blood sugar went: The lower the glucose, the more adrenalin secretion. Moreover, 192 persons undergoing glucose tolerance tests showed no relationship between the appearance of symptoms and the rate of descent of the glucose level.[8] There is thus no reason to believe the rate of decline of glucose levels within the normal range accounts for symptoms popularly attributed to idiopathic reactive hypoglycemia.

To summarize the facts about the controversial subject of idiopathic reactive hypoglycemia: Although many people experience symptoms after eating, most of them have nothing wrong with their blood glucose. In those who do have abnormally low blood sugar after eating, a known cause of reactive hypoglycemia can usually be identified. Properly documented cases of abnormally low blood sugar of unknown cause after eating are very uncommon.

[9] R. A. DeFronzo, R. Hendler, and N. Christensen, *Diabetes* 29 (1980), 125.

[10] R. A. DeFronzo et al., *Diabetes* 26 (1977), 445.

[11] A. J. Garber et al., *Journal of Clinical Investigation* 58 (1976), 7.

[12] J. V. Santiago et al., *Journal of Clinical Endocrinology and Metabolism* 51 (1980), 877.

2. *DRUGS THAT WORK THROUGH INSULIN*

Several of the medications used in the treatment of diabetes mellitus lower blood sugar by stimulating the pancreas to secrete more insulin. These drugs include chlorpropamide (sold as Diabinese), tolbutamide (sold as Orinase), acetohexamide (sold as Dymelor), tolazamide (sold as Tolinase), glipizide (sold as Glucatrol), and glyburide (sold as Diabeta or Micronase). Numerous drugs of this type are coming to market as pharmaceutical companies compete to provide better treatment for diabetes. These drugs are known as "oral hypoglycemic agents" or "oral hypoglycemics" because they are taken by mouth and lower blood glucose. In addition to stimulating insulin secretion, some of these drugs may also increase the sensitivity of body tissues to insulin, so that any given amount of insulin becomes more effective in lowering blood sugar. In either case, insulin mediates the hypoglycemic action of the drugs.

In excessive amounts, these drugs produce severe and prolonged hypoglycemia. As described in Chapter 2, one of the drugs, chlorpropamide, caused devastating brain damage to the drug addict who bought them thinking they were "blue codeines."

Oral hypoglycemics can accumulate in the body when the liver or the kidneys are diseased. Kidney disease, for example, can lead to a buildup of chlorpropamide, tolazamide, or acetohexamide in anyone taking these drugs. Since the kidneys normally excrete them in the urine, these drugs stay in the body when the kidneys fail. The effect is equivalent to taking an increased dose of the drug and can lead to severe hypoglycemia. The same problems can arise when liver disease occurs in a diabetic patient taking one of the drugs inactivated in the liver such as tolbutamide, tolazamide, and acetohexamide. As the drugs build up in the body, their effects intensify and the blood sugar falls.

When taken with oral hypoglycemics, certain other medications increase the potency of the hypoglycemic agents by interfering with the mechanisms that normally inactivate them. The list of drugs that can interfere with these mechanisms is long. It includes many antibiotics (especially the sulfas and the tetracylines), drugs used for arthritis (including aspirin, phenylbutazone, allopurinol, and probenecid), and drugs used to lower blood cholesterol levels (such as clofibrate). For example, a diabetic patient taking oral hypoglycemics may suddenly develop hypoglycemia when treated with antibiotics for a urine infection or with anticoagulant drugs for blood clots.

3. *OTHER DRUGS*

Pentamidine used to be the only effective treatment for a dangerous kind of pneumonia (pneumocystis carinii). About 100 cases of hypoglycemia have been recognized and published as side effects of pentamidine therapy. Pentamidine causes hypoglycemia by releasing insulin from the islet cells in the pancreas. In doing so, however, the pentamidine destroys those insulin-producing cells. The hypoglycemia is therefore temporary, and if enough insulin-producing cells are destroyed, the final result can be *high* blood sugar (diabetes mellitus) because of insulin deficiency. About 30 cases of diabetes mellitus have been reported following pentamidine-induced hypoglycemia. The availability of other effective treatments for pneumocystis carinii pneumonia now avoids these side effects.

Aspirin overdose, especially severe cases in children, can cause hypoglycemia. The means by which aspirin and related drugs lower blood sugar is not known, but they appear to act in some people like oral hypoglycemic agents. Hypoglycemia from aspirin is rare in adults, and it never arises from the low doses usually recommended for pain relief.

Adrenalin-blocking drugs ("beta-blockers") enjoy wide use in the treatment of high blood pressure, irregular heartbeat, glaucoma, and migraine heachaches. They rarely cause hypoglycemia. When they do it's in combination with some other predisposing factor such as alcohol intake or kidney failure. The main concern regarding these drugs is that when given to diabetics taking *other* hypoglycemic medications (such as insulin) they can prevent the shakiness and rapid heartbeat that are often the first warning signs of hypoglycemia. They may also interfere with recovery from hypoglycemia by blocking some of the effects of adrenalin on glycogen breakdown and insulin secretion.

Scantily documented reports have implicated many other drugs as possible causes of hypoglycemia. The strongest cases can probably be made for disopyramide (sold as Norpace) and perhexiline maleate (sold in France as Pexid.). Both are used as treatments for heart conditions. The reports of other drugs causing low blood sugar are so fragmentary and circumstantial, however, that final judgment must await further scientific studies.

4. *UNRIPE ACKEE FRUIT*

Doesn't that sound like something out of *Alice in Wonderland*? Actually, it's something out of Jamaica, where ackee fruit grows abundantly and is a dietary staple. When ripe, ackee fruit is harmless, but if eaten before it ripens can cause a deadly disease known as "Jamaican vomiting sickness." Victims complain of abdominal pain, vomiting, and weakness. Their blood sugar often drops very low—so low that coma, convulsions, and death may occur. The cause of the hypoglycemia is a poison in the unripe fruit known as "hypoglycin." Hypoglycin interferes with gluconeogenesis, and consequently causes hypoglycemia only when glycogen stores have been depleted. Thus, well-nourished individuals who have plenty of glycogen stored in the liver are much less likely to suffer severe hypoglycemia than the malnourished Jamaican who, out of hunger and desperation, eats the fruit before it ripens.

5. *ALCOHOL*

Like unripe ackee fruit, alcohol blocks gluconeogenesis. It causes hypoglycemia in people who haven't recently eaten and who therefore have no food being absorbed from the intestine and no glycogen left in the liver. Such people must rely on the production of new glucose, which alcohol stops. Mrs. Tippler (Chapter 6) had a case of alcohol-induced hypoglycemia. Hers was a case of fasting alcoholic hypoglycemia, which is the most common variety, and the most widely recognized by physicians. Alcohol also causes hypoglycemia in other settings, such as after exercise. When taken with sugar on an empty stomach, it can produce reactive hypoglycemia, as explained earlier in this chapter.

Alcoholic hypoglycemia is a frequent, and easily overlooked, cause of brain malfunction, especially among chronic alcoholics who eat poorly. Police may take such people to the "drunk tank" to sober up. Family and friends may attribute to alcohol rather than hypoglycemia the patient's symptoms of confusion, uncoordination, or coma. The patient himself is usually too tipsy to figure out what's happening. Even a doctor might mistake hypoglycemic seizures for "rum fits," a nickname for convulsions in the alcohol-withdrawal syndrome known as delirium tremens ("the DTs"). Fortunately, most physicians realize that alcohol can alter brain function via hypoglycemia, as well as through its own toxic effect on the nervous system.

6. *INTERNALLY PRODUCED SUBSTANCES THAT ACT LIKE INSULIN*

a) Tumors

Certain large tumors reduce blood glucose levels below normal. Part of this effect arises from outflow of glucose from the bloodstream into the tumor itself, which may consume large amounts of glucose. Recent evidence indicates that such tumors also produce a substance that mimics the action of insulin. This substance increases glucose outflow to tissues all over the body, and blocks glucose input by restraining glycogen breakdown and gluconeogenesis.

b) Antibodies to Insulin Receptors

In order to lower blood sugar, insulin must attach itself to the various tissues of the body. This attachment occurs at specific sites known as "insulin receptors." Like a key in a lock, insulin fits into a receptor and triggers the processes within cells that reduce blood sugar. In the same way that other devices, used by thieves and locksmiths, can also fit a lock and trigger the opening of a door, substances other than insulin can fit into the insulin receptor and trigger the processes that lower blood sugar. Some of these substances are made by tumors, as mentioned above. Antibodies are also capable of attaching to insulin receptors and lowering the level of blood sugar.

Antibodies usually attach themselves to foreign substances such as bacteria and viruses. As part of the body's defenses, antibodies make it easier for killer cells to destroy these invaders. In rare cases, however, the body's defenses turn against its own tissues and build antibodies that attach to its own cells. When these antibodies attach to the thyroid gland, for example, they can make it underactive or overactive. When they attach to insulin receptors, they can cause hypoglycemia. The correction of this rare, and only recently discovered, cause of hypoglycemia consists of giving cortisone, which interferes with antibody production and also opposes the actions of insulin.

c) Antibodies to Insulin

Doctors in Japan have reported a few cases of hypoglycemia in which antibodies bind to insulin itself. Antibodies to insulin are frequently found in people taking insulin. The Japanese cases, however, are not explained by the taking of insulin, and how the antibodies lower blood sugar is not known. The theory is that they bind to and inactivate insulin secreted appropriately after meals, and then release it later when there is no food absorption.

B. LACK OF SUBSTANCES THAT RAISE BLOOD SUGAR

1. *ADRENAL-GLAND FAILURE*

The adrenal glands make two substances that oppose insulin and raise blood sugar. These are cortisol (the natural form of cortisone) and epinephrine (also called adrenalin). As in the case of Enrique Engelhardt in Chapter 1, lack of these substances, due to disease or destruction of the adrenal glands, can cause hypoglycemia.

Adrenal-gland failure is known as Addison's disease. ("Adrenal insufficiency" is another term applied to the same condition.) Typical symptoms include darkening skin color, nausea, weight loss, poor appetite, and blood pressure so low that the sufferer feels faint when standing up. The diagnosis of Addison's disease requires blood tests that document cortisol deficiency. It cannot be diagnosed by hair clippings. Its treatment requires some form of cortisone. Crude extracts of animal adrenal glands will not suffice. Since cortisone treatment can cause serious side effects if given in the wrong dosage, the diagnosis and treatment of this rare cause of hypoglycemia should be undertaken with the consultation of a knowledgeable specialist in internal medicine or endocrinology.

2. *PITUITARY-GLAND FAILURE*

Because its hormones affect so many other glands and body processes, the pituitary gland has been called the master control panel for the body's metabolism. Among other substances, the pituitary makes growth hormone, which opposes some of the actions of insulin. Loss of growth hormone can lead to a lowering of blood sugar, especially in children. The pituitary gland also secretes a hormone that controls the part of the adrenal glands that produce cortisol. Cortisol is another anti-insulin hormone. When the pituitary gland is completely destroyed, the adrenal and thyroid glands malfunction, growth ceases, the ovaries and testicles stop making sex hormones, the breasts can no longer produce milk, and the kidneys may lose their ability to retain water. In this grim picture of complete pituitary failure (known as "panhypopituitarism") the lack of growth hormone and cortisol leads to hypoglycemia.

Destruction or malfunction of the pituitary gland need not be complete. Some functions may survive while others fail. When the pituitary is diseased, secretion of growth hormone is one of the first functions to fail. An isolated lack of growth hormone rarely causes hypoglycemia in adults, but can do so in children. In such cases, the stunting of growth offers a clue to why the blood sugar is low.

3. *GLUCAGON DEFICIENCY*

The deficiency of glucagon has not been documented as a definite cause of hypoglycemia. Glucagon does not appear to be as important as insulin in the minute-to-minute regulation of blood sugar in the normal range. It assists, however, in the recovery from hypoglycemia, and is especially important in the recovery from hypoglycemia caused by too much insulin, as in patients overtreated for diabetes mellitus. Some cases of diabetes mellitus involve destruction not only of the islet cells that produce insulin but also of the glucagon-producing cells. When the glucagon-producing cells do not function, diabetics are prone to severe hypoglycemic attacks from their insulin treatment. Thus, glucagon deficiency may play a contributing role in the causation of some cases of hypoglycemia, but by itself probably does not cause hypoglycemia.

C. PROLONGED, SEVERE STARVATION

People who have been previously well nourished can fast for as long as a month without experiencing hypoglycemia. They convert fat and protein to glucose by the process of gluconeogenesis in the liver and kidneys, and thus maintain essential glucose supplies to the brain. Meanwhile, the muscles and brain come to rely on the breakdown of fat for energy, thus minimizing the need for glucose. Eventually, however, the body runs out of fat and protein building blocks, and glucose production fails. Since the brain continues to use glucose, the blood sugar drops as input falls below outflow. Unless some other cause of hypoglycemia is present, however, this does not occur until starvation is quite advanced.

Hypoglycemia that occurs in well-nourished adults after a shorter fast, such as a day or two, defies explanation on the basis of starvation. In such cases, some other specific cause is at work.

D. LIVER FAILURE

The liver plays a central role in maintaining blood glucose levels. The only reason we are able to eat intermittently, rather than having to nibble all the time to maintain glucose input, is that the liver supplies the rest of our body with sugar between meals. Glycogen is stored in the liver, and is broken down into glucose for release as needed. Once stores of glycogen decline, the liver produces new glucose. The liver makes glucose from simple building blocks such as amino acids, glycerol, and lactic acid. When the liver becomes so sick that it can no longer convert these substances to glucose and can no longer release glucose from glycogen, the blood sugar will fall unless sugar is being absorbed from the intestine (or is coming in through an intravenous needle). Consequently, fasting hypoglycemia results from severe liver damage.

It is estimated that as little as 20% of normal liver function is needed to maintain blood glucose levels, so only in severe liver problems is hypoglycemia encountered. The liver damage may be due to any of a number of diseases, such as viral hepatitis, cancer, or alcoholic cirrhosis.

One could argue that almost all causes listed in this chapter, as well as those described in the next chapter, involve a failure of the liver to produce adequate levels of glucose. In a sense this is true, since most causes of hypoglycemia influence blood glucose through their effect on sugar metabolism in the liver. The point of listing liver disease separately is that *anything* that damages the liver severely enough can result in hypoglycemia.

Some people are born with an inherited lack of the liver enzymes necessary for glycogen breakdown and gluconeogenesis. These people usually experience hypoglycemia in childhood. Their disorders will be discussed in the next chapter.

E. KIDNEY FAILURE

Like the liver and the heart, the kidneys are essential for normal function of many other tissues in the body. When the kidneys can no longer excrete waste products, many systems malfunction, including those responsible for maintaining blood sugar. Appetite and food intake decrease. Muscles no longer release amino acids readily, so the liver lacks amino-acid building blocks for gluconeogenesis. A healthy kidney produces new glucose (gluconeogenesis) in prolonged fasting, and this production declines as the kidneys fail. The low blood sugar occasionally seen in patients with chronic kidney disease probably arises from a combination of these factors.

F. SEVERE CONGESTIVE HEART FAILURE

All body tissues depend on the pumping action of the heart. Dependent tissues include the intestines, the muscles, and the liver, all of which are important in glucose metabolism. When the heart is so sick, for example, that the liver lacks sufficient circulation of blood, gluconeogenesis fails and hypoglycemia can result.

G. SEVERE, WIDESPREAD INFECTION

Like heart failure, severe, widespread infection interferes with the function of tissues throughout the body. Again, these tissues include the liver, and failure of gluconeogenesis probably contributes to the occasional case of hypoglycemia seen in the presence of widespread infection.

SUMMARY

This chapter can be summarized as follows:

1. If the blood glucose level is abnormally low, there's a reason for it.
2. Since many complex processes contribute to keeping

blood glucose levels normal, problems that produce hypoglycemia can arise at many points.

3. Blood glucose levels can fall because of increased *outflow* of glucose from the bloodstream, or because of decreased *input* of glucose into the bloodstream, or both. In most actual cases of hypoglycemia, a combination of factors is at work.
4. Insulin, exercise, early pregnancy, and severe infection all accelerate the *outflow* of glucose from the bloodstream.
5. The causes of impaired glucose *input* are numerous and complex. Therefore, the help of an informed, interested physician is needed to diagnose the specific cause of hypoglycemia.
6. Among the many causes of low blood sugar, idiopathic reactive hypoglycemia has been the most widely misdiagnosed.

Before discussing how a physician can accurately diagnose an individual case of hypoglycemia, let's look at hypoglycemia in infancy and childhood. Although anything that lowers blood sugar in adults can also produce hypoglycemia in youngsters, there are additional causes of hypoglycemia that characteristically show up in childhood.

8

What Causes Hypoglycemia in Children?

As in adults, hypoglycemia in children causes both neuroglycopenic and adrenergic symptoms. Unlike adults, however, children may not offer a sophisticated description of what they experience. Excessive adrenalin may make a child jittery, perspire, or have a rapid heartbeat. Insufficient glucose to the brain of a baby may cause listlessness, limpness, abnormal crying, irregular breathing, poor feeding, or convulsions.

As in adults, hypoglycemia in children causes symptoms that are not unique to low blood sugar. The symptoms should alert parents and physicians to the possibility of hypoglycemia, but alternative explanations such as infection should also be considered. The diagnosis of hypoglycemia depends on the level of blood sugar drawn at the time of the symptoms in question.

If the blood glucose is 40 mg/dl or less during symptoms, and if the symptoms disappear promptly when measures are taken to raise the sugar level, it is reasonable to conclude the child has hypoglycemia. Once this conclusion has been reached, the next step is to figure out *why*.

Anything that causes hypoglycemia in adults can cause it in a child. This includes all disorders discussed in the last chapter.

Alcohol, for example, can lower blood sugar in a 2-year-old as surely as in his 22-year-old father.

Some childhood causes of hypoglycemia persist throughout life. Occasionally the diagnosis of such a case may be missed in childhood, and made only later, in the adult years. An unfortunate instance of this sort involved a 37-year-old woman with a long history of psychiatric problems. She turned out to have diffuse overgrowth of the islet cells—a condition that causes hypoglycemia in children. Her story is told later in this chapter.

Although some causes of hypoglycemia in childhood persist into adulthood, most do not. Many occur only in childhood at a particular stage. We shall consider them in the chronological order of the ages at which they typically arise, as outlined in Table 3.

Table 3

CAUSES OF HYPOGLYCEMIA CHARACTERISTICALLY OCCURRING IN CHILDREN

I. *TEMPORARY HYPOGLYCEMIA IN NEWBORNS*
   A. PREMATURITY
   B. PROBLEMS ACQUIRED THROUGH THE UMBILICAL CORD
      1. *FETAL MALNUTRITION*
      2. *DRUGS*
      3. *DIABETES IN THE MOTHER*
      4. *ERYTHROBLASTOSIS FETALIS*
   C. BECKWITH-WIEDEMANN SYNDROME
II. *PERSISTENT HYPOGLYCEMIA*
   A. SEVERE DISEASES INVOLVING MANY BODY SYSTEMS
      1. *CONGENITAL HEART DISEASE*
      2. *SEVERE, WIDESPREAD INFECTION*
      3. *STARVATION*
      4. *ASPHYXIATION AND THE RESPIRATORY DISTRESS SYNDROME*
      5. *OTHER (CALCIUM DEFICIENCY, BRAIN DAMAGE, MULTIPLE DEFORMITIES)*
   B. SEVERE LIVER DISEASE
   C. EXCESS INSULIN
      1. *DISCRETE TUMOR (INSULINOMA)*
      2. *DIFFUSE OVERGROWTH OF ISLET CELLS*
   D. DEFICIENT ANTI-INSULIN HORMONES
      1. *PITUITARY DISEASE*
      2. *LARON DWARFS*
      3. *ADRENAL-GLAND DISEASE*
   E. INHERITED ENZYME DEFECTS
III. *SPECIAL PROBLEMS OF TODDLERS AND OLDER CHILDREN*
   A. POISONINGS
   B. KETOTIC HYPOGLYCEMIA OF CHILDHOOD

You don't need to digest the material in Table 3 at this point. It is included here as a road map, to show you the territory we will cover in this chapter. If you get lost along the way, you can refer back to it and find your way.

I. TEMPORARY HYPOGLYCEMIA IN NEWBORNS

The newborn child is especially liable to develop low blood sugar. In the first place, glucose *outflow* from the bloodstream is rapid because the brain is six times larger, compared to the rest of the body, in infancy than in adulthood. You will recall that the brain must have glucose at all times, and consumes more of this fuel than does any other tissue. Moreover, the liver, which must supply glucose, is relatively smaller at that age than in the adult. In terms of body proportions, then, the newborn is set more to consume than to produce glucose.

When a baby is born, there is no food in the intestines to be absorbed. All nourishment has been coming to the fetus through the umbilical cord. As soon as the cord is clamped off at birth, therefore, the newborn must rely on glycogen breakdown and gluconeogenesis for *input* of glucose into the bloodstream. If glycogen stores are not well supplied, or if the liver enzymes necessary for liberating glucose from glycogen are not present, mature, and ready to function, hypoglycemia can result.

A newborn infant with no glycogen in its liver must either nurse immediately or rely on the production of new glucose through gluconeogenesis. Unfortunately, some newborns cannot achieve gluconeogenesis, which is a complex process requiring the coordinated function of many enzymes in several tissues. Moreover, many infants are not fed promptly and successfully. As you can see, with Murphy's Law in full force, the baby's blood sugar has ample opportunity to drop.

The frequency of hypoglycemia in newborns is not well known, but it is unquestionably true that hypoglycemia occurs more often within the first 72 hours of life than during any other period. Experts estimate that 14,000 newborn babies suffer hypoglycemia each year in the United States alone.[1] Other experts, with less stringent definitions of hypoglycemia, would put the figure much higher.

[1] **R. L. Gutberlet and M. Cornblath, *Pediatrics* 58 (1976), 10.**

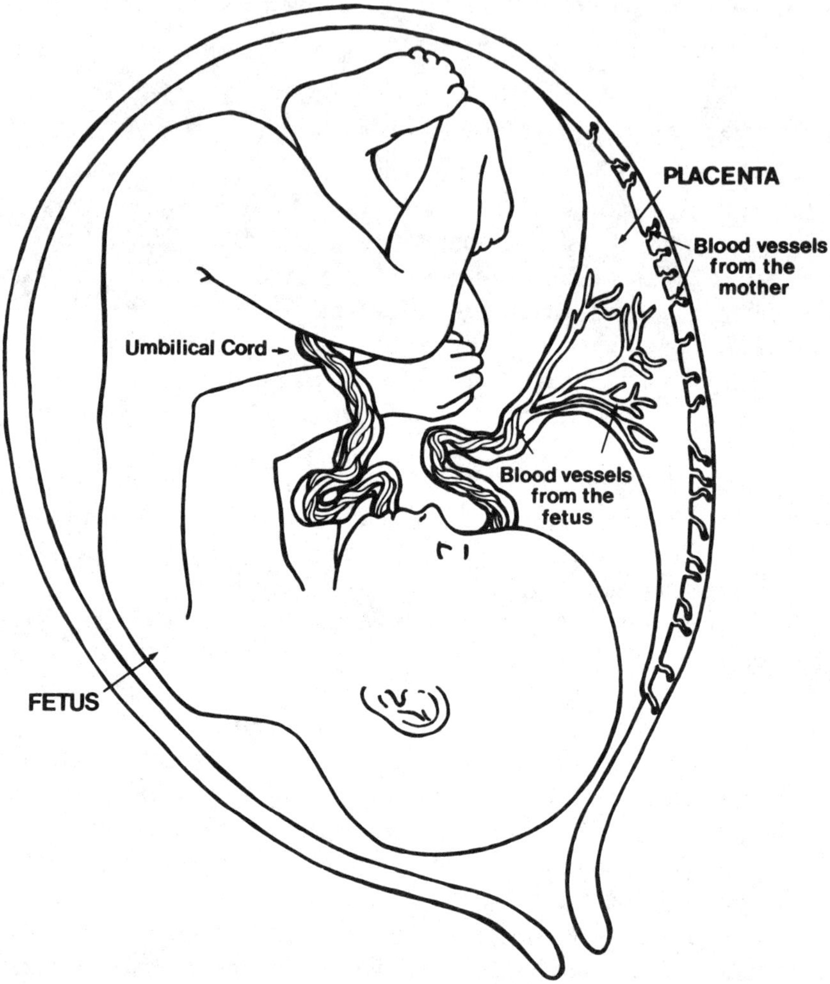

Fig. 11. The fetus within its mother's uterus is nourished through the umbilical cord. The placenta transfers glucose and other nutrients from the mother's circulation to the baby's via the cord. Drugs and antibodies in the mother's bloodstream also get to the fetus by way of the placenta and umbilical cord.

A. PREMATURITY

During its last few weeks in the uterus, a normal fetus accumulates lots of glycogen in its liver. This glycogen stands the newborn in good stead, providing a ready reservoir of glucose to be liberated into the bloodstream as needed. The *premature* infant, however, leaves the uterus before it has had a chance to complete this stocking-up process. Because it enters the world with a smaller supply of liver glycogen, the premature newborn is more liable than a full-term baby to run low on sugar unless it nurses promptly and regularly. Unfortunately, many premature newborns don't nurse well.

Frequently in the premature infant the liver enzymes which carry out the breakdown of glycogen and the manufacture of new glucose are not yet fully ready to function. Until these enzymes develop, the baby will have difficulty maintaining adequate levels of glucose between feedings. Without adequate glucose input, the bloodstream becomes depleted.

B. PROBLEMS ACQUIRED THROUGH THE UMBILICAL CORD

Inside the uterus, the fetus is connected to its mother by the umbilical cord and placenta, as shown in Fig. 11. The placenta transfers nutrients and oxygen from the mother's circulation to the fetus. Since sugar flows freely across the placenta, the fetus will never have hypoglycemia unless the mother does. Once born, however, the baby can develop hypoglycemia from what has previously arrived, or hasn't arrived, from its mother via the cord.

1. *FETAL MALNUTRITION*

Fetal malnutrition results in a small, thin baby. "Small for dates" or "small for gestational age" are other names for this condition, in which the fetus is smaller than normal even though it may have spent a full nine months in the uterus. Since the fetus relies entirely on the placenta and umbilical cord for nourishment from its mother, diseases and malnutrition of the mother and diseases of the placenta can result in a scrawny little fetus. In addition, when twins share the same placenta, one of them may get the "lion's share" of the nutrients, while the other is malnourished. For unknown reasons, malnourished newborn boys are more susceptible to hypoglycemia than girls of similar size and age.

The exact causes of hypoglycemia in these "small for dates" infants are probably several. They have little glycogen stored in the liver to act as a reserve supply of glucose after birth. They may not nurse very well. Their lack of fat (due to undernutrition in the uterus) leaves them unable to switch over successfully to reliance on fat instead of glucose as an energy source. Unable to use much fat for energy, they must rely on glucose and consequently have an accelerated rate of glucose outflow from the bloodstream.[2] In addition, because their bodies are so thin their brains are disproportionately even larger than in normal babies, further taxing the ability of glucose input to keep up with outflow. Some of these babies lack the normal adrenalin response to hypoglycemia to help them get their blood sugar back up to normal.[3] As in the case of premature babies, the liver in these "small for dates" infants may lack the enzymes necessary to produce new glucose through gluconeogenesis.

2. *DRUGS*

Drugs, such as those discussed in Chapter 7, can travel from mother to fetus through the cord, then cause hypoglycemia within a few hours after birth. Alcohol is a prime example of such a drug. Alcohol was formerly given to prevent premature labor. Then, if it failed to stop labor, the premature baby came out drunk, and prone to hypoglycemia.

One particularly troublesome type of drug is still used to stop labor. To prevent a woman from delivering a premature baby, doctors will sometimes administer ritodrine or terbutaline, which stop the uterus from contracting. If this attempt to delay the baby's expulsion from the uterus fails, however, the effects of these drugs on the baby can cause hypoglycemia. These drugs stimulate insulin secretion from the fetal pancreas, and trigger the breakdown of glycogen from the liver. Thus the baby, born after several hours of exposure to these drugs in the uterus, may begin life with both a high level of insulin in the blood and a low reserve of glycogen in the liver. Within an hour such a baby is very likely to show signs of hypoglycemia.

[2] **R. de Leeuw and I. de Vries, *Pediatrics* 58 (1976), 18.**
[3] **L. Stern, T. L. Sourkes, and N. Ratha, *Biologia Neonatorum* 11 (1967) 129.**

Oral hypoglycemia medications (given to the mother for treatment of diabetes) can cross into the baby's circulation and cause severe, prolonged hypoglycemia in the newborn. For this reason they should not be used to treat diabetes in pregnant women.

3. *DIABETES IN THE MOTHER*

Diabetes mellitus, a condition in which blood glucose levels are elevated, is common during pregnancy. Many women whose blood sugar levels are otherwise normal will develop diabetes during the late stages of pregnancy. Glucose, abundant in the mother's bloodstream, crosses the placenta in increased amounts and stimulates the fetal pancreas to secrete a great deal of insulin. The insulin-producing tissues of the pancreas enlarge. As the cord is cut, the flood of sugar from the mother stops abruptly, but insulin continues temporarily to pour forth from the baby's pancreas, driving down the glucose level. The higher the mother's level of blood glucose, the greater is the tendency for the baby to develop hypoglycemia after birth. Careful control of the mother's blood sugar prior to delivery, so that the fetus is exposed only to normal levels of blood glucose, prevents this problem.

4. *ERYTHROBLASTOSIS FETALIS*

Erythroblastosis fetalis is the name given to a condition in which antibodies from the mother cross the placenta and destroy the red blood cells of the baby. This occurs especially when the mother has an Rh-negative blood type and the fetus has inherited an Rh-positive blood type from its father. The process usually begins during the birth of an Rh-positive child to an Rh-negative mother. During the trauma of childbirth some of the baby's blood cells enter the mother's circulation and sensitize her system against Rh-positive cells. Then, during *subsequent* pregnancies involving Rh-positive babies, the mother makes antibodies against Rh-positive cells. These antibodies cross the placenta and attack the fetal blood cells.

Babies born with this syndrome are usually very ill, and hypoglycemia is only one of their problems. The low blood sugar seems to be caused by high levels of insulin in the baby's circulation, but the reasons why the baby's pancreas oversecretes insulin are not known. Like the infants of diabetic mothers, these babies have temporary enlargement of the insulin-producing cells of the pancreas.

Treatment of erythroblastosis fetalis often involves bleeding the baby and replacing its own blood with transfusions, in order to rid the bloodstream of the attacking antibodies from the mother. This maneuver is called "exchange transfusion." If carried out with blood to which the usual anticoagulant solution has been added, the hypoglycemia may worsen after the transfusion. This is because most blood for transfusion is mixed with a sugary solution of citric acid to keep it from clotting. The high sugar content of the transfused blood further stimulates the overenthusiastic insulin secretion, and a downward rebound of the blood sugar results. Physicians can prevent this problem by slowly administering intravenous glucose after the transfusion, or else by using blood to which excess glucose has not been added.

Medical scientists have devised a means to prevent an Rh-negative mother from becoming sensitized to the Rh-positive cells of her offspring. It involves giving the mother an injection of antibodies shortly after childbirth, to take the fetal blood cells out of her circulation before they can trigger the immune response. This advance in medical science is making erythroblastosis fetalis an increasingly rare problem.

C. BECKWITH-WIEDEMANN SYNDROME

Babies with this syndrome typically have large bodies, a large tongue, and an abnormal navel. Most of them have abnormal creases of the earlobes, and many have a birthmark on the upper part of the face. A variety of tissues throughout the body are enlarged, including the insulin-producing cells of the pancreas. High levels of insulin in the bloodstream cause hypoglycemia in at least half of these babies. The hypoglycemia appears in the first week of life, and may last several days before subsiding on its own. The cause of this unusual condition is not known.

All of the causes of hypoglycemia described above are self-limited: The blood sugar will eventually return to normal on its own without specific treatment other than supplying the baby with enough nourishment by mouth or vein. The premature or malnourished infant will grow and mature; drugs and antibodies from the mother's circulation will eventually dissipate even without specific treatment. Thus, the hypoglycemia they cause will be only temporary. We shall next discuss causes of low blood sugar in newborns and children that persist until the underlying disorder is specifically corrected.

II. PERSISTENT HYPOGLYCEMIA

A. SEVERE DISEASES INVOLVING MANY BODY SYSTEMS

As in adults, diseases that disrupt the function of many vital organs can cause hypoglycemia.

1. *CONGENITAL HEART DISEASE*

Heart disease, for example, can prevent the liver from achieving gluconeogenesis as surely in a baby as in an adult. In babies, severe heart disease is usually due to a congenital deformity of the heart or major blood vessels. In many such instances, the blood does not contain sufficient oxygen, so the baby looks blue. These "blue babies" are liable to have hypoglycemia until the underlying circulatory disorder is corrected, usually by surgery.

2. *SEVERE, WIDESPREAD INFECTION*

Severe, widespread infection is even more likely to cause hypoglycemia in a child than an adult. We covered this topic in the previous chapter.

3. *STARVATION*

Starvation brings on hypoglycemia much more quickly in newborns than in adults. This can be a problem particularly if the baby has to have an operation. It was previously customary to withhold feeding from little babies for hours before an operation, in order to reduce the chance of vomiting. Now it is recognized that the newborn baby needs extra nutrition to cope with the stress and energy demands of surgery, and efforts are made to supply glucose by mouth or by vein to prevent starvation, which leads so quickly to hypoglycemia in the newborn.

4. *ASPHYXIATION AND THE RESPIRATORY DISTRESS SYNDROME*

Asphyxiation, or lack of oxygen, can be a severe problem at the time of childbirth, as the infant emerges from the birth canal and tries to take its first breaths of air. Especially if the umbilical cord has been pinched off during delivery, the baby's tissues may be starved for oxygen and unable to function properly. All body processes, including those that supply glucose to the circulation, can fail in such circumstances. A common variant of this problem is the "respiratory distress syndrome."

Infant respiratory distress syndrome is especially common in babies who already have increased risk of hypoglycemia for other reasons, discussed above, such as prematurity, infection, or a diabetic mother. Their tendency to hypoglycemia is compounded by the respiratory distress syndrome, in which the lungs have difficulty supplying enough oxygen to the bloodstream. The distressed infant, starved for oxygen, struggles to breathe. The increased muscular exertion drains glucose and ketones from its bloodstream, and the lack of oxygen impairs glucose input. Hypoglycemia can thus be a feature of newborn respiratory distress syndrome, and improves as the lungs do.

5. *OTHER (CALCIUM DEFICIENCY, BRAIN DAMAGE, MULTIPLE DEFORMITIES)*

Other problems in the newborn affecting many body tissues and often leading to hypoglycemia include low blood calcium level, multiple congenital deformities, and brain damage. The symptoms of these conditions can mimic those of hypoglycemia, so the physician must be on the alert to test for hypoglycemia in these situations and to give glucose if needed.

B. SEVERE LIVER DISEASE

Liver disease of any cause, if severe enough, can of course cause hypoglycemia, since the liver is the source of glucose (from glycogen and gluconeogenesis), which prevents blood sugar from falling between feedings.

C. EXCESS INSULIN

As explained in the preceding chapters, insulin is the most powerful single influence bringing down the level of blood sugar. It blocks input of glucose into the bloodstream, and it speeds outflow of glucose into the tissues. It also accelerates the delivery of other nutrients into body tissues, and thus promotes growth and weight gain. Consequently, most children with hypoglycemic conditions characterized by excessive amounts of insulin are big for their age.

1. *DISCRETE TUMOR (INSULINOMA)*

Discrete tumors of the islet cells that produce insulin are called insulinomas. They can occur in adults or children, and were discussed in the previous chapter. They cause hypoglycemia by secreting too much insulin. In children they are usually part of an inherited syndrome involving tumors of the pancreas, the pituitary, and the parathyroid glands. A family history of such tumors should alert the physician to the possibility of insulinoma in a child.

2. *DIFFUSE OVERGROWTH OF ISLET CELLS*

If this book had been written ten years ago, a number of distinct and different conditions all involving overgrowth of insulin-producing cells in the pancreas would have been listed here. Some would have been called "leucine sensitivity" and others "nesidioblastosis." Now, however, it is clear that these conditions overlap one another to a great extent. They all involve diffuse enlargement and overactivity of the insulin-producing cells in the pancreas. There are probably several causes of this sort of condition, and some cases run in families, while others do not.

In all of these cases, hypoglycemia results from excessive amounts of insulin pouring forth from the pancreas. Blood tests show low blood sugar with inappropriately high insulin levels, as in cases of insulin-producing tumors. The search for a tumor, however, turns up none. When an operation is done to look for a tumor of the pancreas, and a portion of the pancreas is removed, microscopic examination shows diffuse overgrowth of the insulin-producing cells. Some of the patterns seen under the microscope resemble the appearance of the normal pancreas in a fetus, before the hormone-producing cells have clustered neatly together into nests, or "islets." Others look fairly normal except for enlargement of the islet cells.

The term "leucine sensitivity" was formerly applied to some of these cases because dietary intake of the amino acid leucine stimulates a massive outpouring of insulin, with severe hypoglycemia after eating. I saw a case of this in an American Indian boy with a history of mental retardation and seizures. A diet restricted in leucine had been prescribed, but this was virtually impossible to follow while living on a reservation, where pinto beans (which have a high content of leucine) are eaten more than any other food. Although impossible to prove in retrospect, it is probable that his mental retardation and seizure disorder were the result of brain damage from prolonged hypoglycemia in early childhood. Like some other cases, this boy's tendency to hypoglycemia lessened over the years so that the need for dietary restriction became less. Unfortunately, however, his mental retardation was permanent.

Leucine sensitivity characterizes many of the cases now lumped together as nesidioblastosis, or diffuse islet-cell overgrowth. Some of these cases respond well to restriction of dietary foodstuffs containing leucine. In others, administration of anti-insulin hormones, such as glucagon (combined with zinc, to make it long-acting), or cortisone is necessary. Drugs that block the secretion of insulin from the pancreas have been used with some success also. In many cases, however, surgical removal of the pancreas, or at least a large portion of it, is necessary to reduce the secretion of insulin enough to stop the hypoglycemia. Surgery was the treatment used for the 37-year-old with diffuse islet-cell overgrowth mentioned at the start of this chapter, whose diagnosis was evidently overlooked for years. Her story, which follows, illustrates that (1) the symptoms of hypoglycemia are not specific, and (2) you must first suspect the possibility of hypoglycemia, then establish that hypoglycemia is present by measuring the blood sugar, then press on to diagnose the specific cause of low blood sugar.

This 37-year-old woman[4] had a long history of psychiatric problems, including paranoid ideas and assaultive behavior dating back to childhood. She had been a patient in more than one psychiatric hospital and had a diagnosis of chronic schizophrenia. Her mother noticed her staggering and confused one day, as if drunk.

[4] **Case Records of the Massachusetts General Hospital (Case 1-1983), *New England Journal of Medicine* 308 (1983), 30.**

Then within ten minutes of eating an orange, she improved. Later, while visiting the psychiatric clinic, she reported feeling sweaty and weak, so a physician checked her glucose level. It was 53 mg/dl, in the borderline, or "gray," zone. The doctor suspected hypoglycemia, so he ordered a five-hour oral glucose tolerance test. It was normal, and she had no symptoms during the test. On another occasion, however, when she was sweaty and couldn't think clearly in the hospital, a doctor alertly ordered a plasma glucose. It was low, at 37 mg/dl. A few days later when she was again confused, her plasma glucose was measured at 32 mg/dl. A corresponding insulin level was higher than expected, suggesting some disorder of the pancreas. At surgery she was found to have diffuse overgrowth of the insulin-producing cells of the pancreas, which characteristically occurs in childhood. One wonders how much of her chronic schizophrenia was really brain malfunction from chronically unrecognized hypoglycemia.

D. DEFICIENT ANTI-INSULIN HORMONES

As in adults, a lack of hormones that oppose the action of insulin on blood sugar can cause hypoglycemia. In children, however, the diseases causing these deficiencies differ from those in adults.

1. *PITUITARY DISEASE*

The pituitary gland secretes growth hormone, which slows the outflow of glucose from the bloodstream and also promotes gluconeogenesis. These two actions help prevent the blood sugar from falling. The pituitary also secretes other hormones that stimulate the thyroid and adrenal glands to put out their respective hormones. Thyroid and adrenal hormones both contribute to normal glucose production, so the combined lack of all pituitary secretions can produce severe hypoglycemia.

The pituitary may lack one of its hormones, such as growth hormone, while the rest of its functions remain intact. In such cases the tendency to hypoglycemia is usually quite mild and the diagnosis may be overlooked for some time until lack of growth becomes obvious. The fetus grows normally within the uterus even without growth hormone from the pituitary gland, because the mother and the placenta provide all the growth-stimulating hormones necessary before birth. A congenital lack of growth hormone, therefore, does not produce a tiny newborn. Only later does the impairment of linear growth become obvious.

When several pituitary hormones are lacking, there are usually more clues that something is amiss. For example, absence of the pituitary gland may occur in association with other congenital deformities. Any of the following abnormalities can provide a clue that the entire pituitary may be absent or diseased: abnormal body size, tiny penis in a baby boy, cleft palate, harelip, and a deformity of the eye that the doctor can see using special instruments.

Besides congenital absence of the pituitary or one of its hormones, other diseases, such as infection or tumor, can destroy a child's pituitary and in this way lead to hypoglycemia. When this occurs, growth hormone is usually one of the first pituitary hormones to fail. The slowing of growth suggests the correct diagnosis.

2. *LARON DWARFS*

A medical scientist named Dr. Laron discovered that certain short individuals who appear to lack the effects of growth hormone actually have high levels of growth hormone in the bloodstream. Their growth hormone, however, is not effective in promoting growth or preventing hypoglycemia. Many of these patients experience low blood sugar. The first suspicion was that these individuals might produce a defective form of growth hormone, but this did not turn out to be true. When injected with normal growth hormone, these people still didn't grow. These observations fit in with previous discoveries that growth hormone does not exert its effects directly. Instead, growth hormone stimulates the liver to produce substances collectively named "somatomedin," and it is the somatomedin that actually stimulates growth and prevents hypoglycemia.

These patients, sometimes referred to as "Laron dwarfs," are suffering from somatomedin deficiency. The liver of a Laron dwarf cannot produce somatomedin even in the presence of plenty of growth hormone. Thus, just like someone with growth hormone deficiency, they are subject to hypoglycemia.

3. *ADRENAL-GLAND DISEASE*

Since adrenal hormones help stimulate glucose production, their absence can cause hypoglycemia. A child's adrenal glands, like an adult's, can be damaged by hemorrhage or infection. In addition, however, congenital diseases affect the adrenal glands.

In the adrenals, as elsewhere, Murphy's Law is at work. Since the production of adrenal hormones requires several steps, each controlled by specific enzymes, there are multiple points of possible breakdown. Medical research has identified several enzyme-deficiency states that prevent the adrenal glands from producing their proper and necessary hormones. Children born with these deficiencies are liable to develop hypoglycemia until accurate diagnosis leads to appropriate treatment with the missing hormones.

Since the adrenal hormones control much more than blood sugar, these infants may have other very serious problems as well, such as low blood pressure, low blood sodium, and abnormal development of the genitals. These associated abnormalities point the physician toward the correct diagnosis.

E. INHERITED ENZYME DEFECTS

Enzymes, as explained in Chapter 6, are essential for proper function of all body tissues, including the adrenals, the liver, the muscles, fat tissue, and every other organ involved in blood glucose regulation. Consequently, as you might expect, there are literally dozens of diseases affecting blood glucose that are due to defective or missing enzymes. A college course in biochemistry would be required in order to understand the details of what is going wrong in each instance, so only the broad outlines will be explained here.

In order to liberate glucose from glycogen, several key enzymes are necessary. Their absence results in a buildup of glycogen in the liver. These conditions are called "glycogen-storage diseases," and the ones that cause hypoglycemia are known as Types I, III, VI and IX.

Even more complex than the breakdown of glycogen is the production of new glucose from other substances within the body. This process of gluconeogenesis involves the conversion of amino acids (building blocks of protein) into glucose, and the derivation of energy from fat metabolism. So numerous are the enzymes involved that many different conditions, each quite rare, cause hypoglycemia through impairment of gluconeogenesis.

Still other enzyme-deficiency conditions cause accumulation of abnormal substances within the liver that interfere with *both* gluconeogenesis and glycogen breakdown and result in severe hypoglycemia.

Not only fasting, but also *reactive* (after-meals) hypoglycemia can be caused by enzyme deficiencies, as in the case of two rare conditions—galactosemia and hereditary fructose intolerance. In these diseases severe hypoglycemia follows the intake of certain sugars—galactose and fructose.

III. SPECIAL PROBLEMS OF TODDLERS AND OLDER CHILDREN

A. POISONINGS

The well-known tendency of toddlers to put things into their mouths creates all sorts of health hazards. Children eat aspirin, oral hypoglycemic drugs, ackee fruit, and alcohol, and develop hypoglycemia just as surely as adults do. Since children are smaller than adults, a smaller dose of the offending substance suffices to lower their blood sugar. This has been a particular problem with alcohol.

Hypoglycemia has been reported in cases of children sponged down with alcohol for fever, and in children who helped their parents clean up after a cocktail party by emptying the glasses. The medicine cabinet has always attracted inquisitive youngsters, and in addition to oral hypoglycemic pills for diabetes, a child may there find his parents' mouthwash available for tasting. Since Cepacol contains 14% alcohol, Scope 18.5%, and Listerine 26.9%, a small child can get enough alcohol from mouthwash to affect his blood glucose.[5]

Prevention of such problems seemed a simple matter to me until I had a few children of my own.

B. KETOTIC HYPOGLYCEMIA OF CHILDHOOD

This rather common form of hypoglycemia affects children between the ages of 18 months and 9 years. Boys are affected more frequently than girls, and the patients are often small and thin.

[5] **E. R. Weller-Fahy, L. W. Berger, and W. G. Troutman, *Pediatrics* 66 (1980), 302.**

Although its cause is still in dispute, extensive studies have taught us a lot about it.

Ketotic hypoglycemia of childhood occurs only during fasting, and indeed seems to consist of an inability to maintain normal gluconeogenesis even though all the necessary hormones are present in appropriate amounts. Since the longest fast is generally overnight, these children typically develop symptoms of hypoglycemia in the early-morning hours. Sunday morning, when breakfast is delayed because the parents are sleeping late, is an especially common time for them to develop headache and irritability because of low blood sugar.

Like normal children, these patients are able to utilize fat, in the form of *ketones* (fat-breakdown products used for fuel by muscle and brain). The presence of these ketones accounts for the name "*ketotic* hypoglycemia," and distinguishes this condition from other diseases in which the body is unable to switch over from glucose to fat as an energy source.

These children are also able to utilize glycogen normally. Moreover, when intravenous amino acids and glycerol are given, these patients can convert them into glucose through gluconeogenesis. The problem seems to be that amino acids, especially *alanine,* which is probably the most important single building block used for glucose manufacture in the fasting state, are not present in the bloodstream in normal amounts. They are thus not available to the liver for gluconeogenesis. Why the muscles do not release alanine normally into the bloodstream is not understood. Cortisone treatment improves the release of alanine from muscle, and in this way corrects the problem. Rather than a cortisone pill at bedtime, however, the preferred treatment is simply frequent feedings of starchy foods.

It has been suggested that the reason children grow out of this condition by age 9 is that by then they are tall enough to open the refrigerator door by themselves and get a snack when a dropping level of blood glucose makes them hungry. Actually, since we do not know the root cause of the problem in the first place, we don't know why it gets better. In all likelihood, ketotic hypoglycemia results from more than one underlying cause and will be subdivided into more specific disease categories once we learn what is really going on. This applies to other causes of hypoglycemia as well.

This chapter of the book will no doubt be longer in future editions. Many specific details of glucose metabolism in the human body are still only vaguely understood. As future research expands our understanding, diseases now ignored or lumped into catch-all categories will no doubt be defined, and specific, appropriate treatment made available. In glucose metabolism, as in all areas of medicine, what we don't know about the human body still far outweighs what we do.

SUMMARY

To summarize the currently understood causes of hypoglycemia in children:

1. Newborns, particularly those born prematurely or small for gestational age, are prone to suffer hypoglycemia.
2. Most cases of hypoglycemia in the first 72 hours of life are temporary, and resolve without treatment more specific than giving glucose by mouth or by vein.
3. Persistent hypoglycemia in a newborn demands specific diagnosis and therapy to prevent brain damage.
4. Anything that causes hypoglycemia in an adult can also cause it in a child.
5. Certain diseases, such as deficiencies of enzymes needed for glucose production, cause hypoglycemia that typically shows up first in childhood.
6. Toddlers are especially prone to ketotic hypoglycemia of childhood, and to poisonings.
7. Additional causes of hypoglycemia will doubtless be discovered as future research reveals more details of glucose metabolism in humans.

Now that we have reviewed the causes of hypoglycemia, let's turn to the issue of how to figure out which one applies to an individual case. The next chapter will show how you can help your doctor answer the question: If my blood sugar is low, *why* is it low?

9

Finding the Cause of Your Case of Hypoglycemia

The purpose of this chapter is to enable you to comprehend and cooperate with your physician's efforts to find the specific cause of your low blood sugar, should you be a victim of hypoglycemia. It is not meant as a cookbook for you to diagnose yourself. From the two previous chapters you know that we are talking about a technical subject, and that the help of a trained professional is indispensable. This chapter, however, should enable you to understand what your doctor is doing as he seeks to solve your diagnostic puzzle, and to help him succeed.

FIRST THINGS FIRST

Before getting into how to find the specific cause of your case of hypoglycemia, I want to emphasize that the first order of business is to make certain that your blood sugar really is low.

Until you are certain that your symptoms are due to hypoglycemia, and not something else that produces identical symptoms, your attention should be focused on the question of *whether* your blood sugar is low, not *why* it is low. To find out *whether* it is low, your blood sugar must be measured during symptoms, as explained in Chapter 4.

If the laboratory reports your blood glucose to be under 40 mg/dl, or your plasma glucose to be under 45 mg/dl, at the time of your symptoms, and if your symptoms then disappear when your blood sugar is raised, it is highly probable that you do indeed have hypoglycemia. To help exclude possible sources of human error, however, it is a good idea to repeat the measurement during symptoms a second time. Reassurance that accurate laboratory techniques were used to measure the blood glucose (as discussed in Chapter 3) would also be helpful.

If your plasma glucose was not definitely low during symptoms, but was instead in the "gray zone" of 45–60 mg/dl, it becomes doubly important to ascertain whether hypoglycemia is really the problem, before launching into the search for causes of hypoglycemia. To be sure that glucose levels in the gray zone are responsible for your symptoms, you must repeatedly measure the blood sugar during symptoms and also show that raising the blood sugar eliminates the symptoms.

The search for a specific cause of hypoglycemia will cost you time and money. Better be sure you're on the right path before you invest in the journey. Consider the case of Laura.

Laura was a 53-year-old woman with symptoms of shakiness, perspiration, rapid heartbeat, and nervousness. Coffee seemed to make the symptoms worse. During a glucose tolerance test she felt her typical symptoms, and her plasma glucose reached a low point of 50 mg/dl. On the basis of this information, her doctor decided she was hypoglycemic. He ordered tests of her pituitary and adrenal-gland function and kidney and liver function, and measurements of her plasma insulin levels. The total bill was over $300. Unable to reach a specific diagnosis, he referred her to an endocrinologist for further evaluation. Before any more extensive and expensive searching for a cause of hypoglycemia, however, the endocrinologist decided to measure her plasma glucose during spontaneously occurring symptoms. Four such measurements were made, all between 78 and 94 mg/dl. Since her blood sugar was normal during her symptoms, hypoglycemia was obviously not their cause. The doctor searched for other causes of nervousness, perspiration, tremor, and palpitations. He found that Laura's thyroid gland was overactive, and when this was corrected, her symptoms vanished.

Laura's case underscores point number one: First be sure you have hypoglycemia. Not until you are certain that low blood sugar is causing your symptoms is it appropriate to spend time and money looking for the cause of your low blood sugar.

In looking for the cause of hypoglycemia, the first thing your doctor will do is listen to your story. We call this "taking a history." By listening carefully and asking the right questions, a physician can focus in on the most likely possible causes. You can help by observing your symptoms carefully enough to be able to answer the following questions.

TAKING (AND GIVING) THE HISTORY

Would you please describe your symptoms?

Symptoms due to hypoglycemia, though variable from one person to the next, tend to be quite stereotyped and repetitive within the same individual. They are also intermittent rather than constant, because food intake temporarily relieves them.

Some of your symptoms may not be due to low blood sugar. Therefore, it is more important to convey to the doctor what you have been experiencing than it is to explain your theories of what is causing your symptoms. Don't try to give him your interpretations or diagnoses at this point. Too many patients say something like: "Last Saturday night while out with my girlfriend for ice cream, I had an allergic reaction to the pistachio nuts, and then my blood sugar went low and I developed a terrible migraine."

Maybe your blood sugar fell, and maybe it didn't. Maybe it was a migraine headache. Maybe it wasn't. Just tell the doctor what you experienced at the time. Let him proceed from there—that's what he's paid for. Just describe to him the throbbing discomfort in your left cheek and upper molars that started when you bit into the ice cream. It could be an abscessed tooth, or a sinus infection, instead of a migraine.

Similarly, maybe that feeling you had after the pistachio ice cream was an allergic reaction, or maybe it wasn't. If it was, it might have been due to something other than the nuts. Tell him instead what you experienced—rash, swelling, wheezing, itching, diarrhea, whatever. Let him do the diagnosing. The more specifically you can describe your symptoms, the better chance your doctor has to reach an accurate diagnosis.

Does food intake alleviate the symptoms? If so, which foods, and how soon?

Answers to these questions may clarify which of your symptoms are related to low blood sugar and which are not, since raising the blood glucose will promptly relieve most hypoglycemic symptoms. Refined sugar is absorbed most quickly, and therefore relieves hypoglycemic symptoms most promptly.

What seems to bring on, or provoke, an attack of symptoms?

Exercise, alcohol, medications, skipping a meal, certain foods—each can affect the blood sugar in a different way and point to one or another cause of hypoglycemia. The observant patient can thus provide the physician with key information that may lead toward the correct diagnosis.

Do your symptoms occur only while fasting (such as in the morning before breakfast), or only after eating, or both?

With this question the doctor is trying to distinguish between *fasting* and *reactive* hypoglycemia, as explained in Chapter 7.

Symptoms that occur *only* after eating point to the very few entities that cause exclusively reactive hypoglycemia. Many disorders, such as insulinoma or pituitary failure, typically produce fasting hypoglycemia, but can sometimes cause reactive hypoglycemia as well. Other disorders, such as ketotic hypoglycemia of childhood, explained in Chapter 8, occur only while fasting.

It is useful to give a detailed account of the timing of meals in relation to symptoms. Some people eat nothing between supper at 6:00 P.M. and breakfast at 8:00 A.M. (and thus endure a 14-hour fast every day); others have a midnight snack every night and never go more than six hours without food.

Have any of your blood relatives had hypoglycemia?

This information might point toward inherited causes of hypoglycemia, such as enzyme defects and some forms of insulin-secreting tumors. Unfortunately, however, so many people have been erroneously diagnosed as having hypoglycemia that a positive answer is of little value unless accompanied by the specific cause of the hypoglycemia, such as insulinoma.

Has your weight been increasing or decreasing?

The many causes of hypoglycemia that work through insulin, or through insulin-like substances, tend to produce weight gain. This is because insulin moves glucose and the building blocks of fat and protein from the bloodstream into the tissues. Consequently, the tissues enlarge. Insulin is thus a "body builder." On the other hand, deficiency of adrenal hormones tends to cause weight loss.

Although insulin excess and adrenal-hormone deficiency each cause hypoglycemia, they have opposite effects on body weight. The answer to the above question, therefore, can guide the investigation toward or away from either of these entities.

Many questions in the taking of a history are aimed at specific causes of hypoglycemia. Into this category fall such questions as:

1. How much alcohol do you drink, and of what kinds, and in what relation to meals, exercise, and symptoms?
2. What medications do you take?
3. Have you had any liver disease or kidney disorder?
4. Have you ever had stomach surgery for ulcers?
5. Have you had a cancer or a tumor?

The importance of the above questions will be obvious to any reader who has digested Chapters 6, 7, and 8.

6. Are your menstrual periods regular?

Normal menstruation would be strong evidence against pituitary disease. In a man, a normal level of sexual interest and potency would provide similar evidence of normal pituitary-gland function.

7. Have you noticed any change in skin color?

Adrenal-gland failure and severe liver disease each have their own characteristic effects here.

8. Have you noticed loss of appetite, a dizzy or faint feeling when standing, a craving for salt, or loss of armpit or pubic hair (in a woman)?

These symptoms could point to adrenal disease. They are *not sufficient* evidence to make a diagnosis of adrenal-gland failure, however. Like all aspects of the history, they point the way toward a possible diagnosis, but biochemical proof of adrenal insufficiency must be obtained before long-term treatment is prescribed. Just as the symptoms of hypoglycemia are nonspecific, so are the symptoms of the diseases that cause it.

Many other questions will arise in the course of giving a history. Each elicits details of various symptoms and helps the doctor include or exclude diagnostic possibilities from consideration. Once the history has been taken, it is time to examine the patient.

EXAMINING THE PATIENT

In adults with hypoglycemia, physical examination seldom adds much information to what has already been learned from a careful history. In a newborn child, on the other hand, where the only available history is from the mother and the obstetrician, physical examination is often very helpful.

In a newborn with hypoglycemia, pituitary disease may be suggested by puffiness, midline congenital deformities, a tiny penis, or an abnormal appearance of the back of the eyes. Ambiguous genitals—neither clearly male nor female—suggest the possibility of an enzyme deficiency blocking the production of cortisol in the adrenal glands. A large baby with a large tongue and a hernia where the umbilical cord inserts into the abdomen may have the Beckwith-Wiedemann syndrome, described in the previous chapter. Small body size without deformity may be diagnostic of fetal malnourishment, which predisposes to temporary hypoglycemia.

In adults, on the other hand, there is usually less to be found during physical examination of a hypoglycemic patient than during the history. Absent pubic and armpit hair in an adult suggests possible adrenal-gland or pituitary-gland deficiency. One looks for scars on the abdomen from previous ulcer surgery, for abnormal skin color, and for tumors large enough to see or feel, but the patient has usually already disclosed such information in his history. The odor of alcohol may belie a history in which drinking was denied or grossly underestimated.

Physical examination gave the clue that lead to the proper diagnosis in the case of a teenager named Luke Lancaster. Luke was in coma at 5:00 o'clock in the morning when brought by ambulance to the emergency room of a hospital near his home. His blood glucose was 15 mg/dl, and he revived after intravenous glucose. He gave a history of diabetes, treated for several years with the same dose of 35 units of slow-acting insulin each morning. A year earlier, Luke had dropped out of medical follow-up care because he didn't like going to the pediatrician's office "with all those little kids in the waiting room." Nevertheless, he stoutly maintained that he had been taking every day the same dose of insulin as always, and had not increased his exercise or decreased his food intake recently.

That history raised the question of *why* 35 units of insulin was now too much for him. Why should that amount of insulin now cause hypoglycemia when it never used to? Physical examination provided the answer.

The emergency-room doctor admitted Luke to the hospital and reduced his dose of insulin to 28 units each morning. The next day Luke had a blood sugar of 27 mg/dl. He had taken *less* insulin than before, had eaten normally, had not been exercising, and yet his blood sugar was again abnormally low. An endocrinologist was consulted and noticed on physical examination that Luke's face was puffy and his complexion was pale. A tap on the heel cord with a reflex hammer showed Luke's reflexes to be slower than normal. These physical findings suggested the possibility of hypothyroidism, which is a deficiency of thyroid hormone caused by disease of the thyroid gland. Specific laboratory tests soon confirmed this suspicion. Luke's body lacked thyroid hormone. This hormone speeds up most body processes, including the breakdown of insulin. Deficient in thyroid hormone, Luke's body no longer destroyed insulin as quickly as before, so insulin was building up in his body and causing the blood sugar to fall.

Luke also had other consequences of hypothyroidism, including slow thinking (his grades had been falling), constipation, fatigue, and facial puffiness. Treatment with thyroid hormone pills solved all these problems. Once his body tissues were receiving the proper amount of thyroid hormone, they destroyed insulin at a normal rate again, and he once again needed the full 35 units, or more, of insulin each day to control his diabetes.

History and physical examination usually do not suffice to pinpoint the cause of hypoglycemia. As in Luke's case, laboratory tests are usually needed. What was learned in the history and physical examination should of course influence the choice of which tests are used, and which ones may reasonably be omitted. Since no single, logical sequence of laboratory tests is necessary for all cases of hypoglycemia, let's discuss the thinking and strategy behind those most often employed.

LABORATORY TESTING

It is helpful to distinguish the types of hypoglycemia that occur *only after eating* (reactive hypoglycemia) from those that may occur also in the *fasting* state. The list of diseases that cause hypoglycemia only after food intake is fairly short. It includes previous stomach surgery, galactosemia, hereditary fructose intolerance, "idiopathic" reactive hypoglycemia, alcohol intake with sugar, and large doses of sugar such as the glucose tolerance test. The age of the patient, the history, and a few blood tests will help sort out these possibilities in short order.

On the other hand, if hypoglycemia occurs *fasting,* whether or not the blood sugar also falls following food intake, the list of possible causes is long. Moreover, among the causes of fasting hypoglycemia are conditions that can seriously threaten the life or health of the patient. It is thus very helpful to know whether the patient's blood sugar will fall abnormally low during a fast. A good way to start the laboratory evaluation of the patient, then, is to fast the patient long enough to produce hypoglycemia. In a baby this may take only four to six hours. An adult may require a 72-hour fast, followed by exercise, though less will usually suffice.

During the fast, the patient should be watched carefully for symptoms of hypoglycemia so that treatment to raise the blood sugar can be given promptly, as soon as blood has been drawn for glucose and other tests. By intentionally letting the patient become briefly hypoglycemic during an observed fast, the doctor accomplishes two very important steps:

1. He finds out whether the patient really has fasting hypoglycemia, and
2. if hypoglycemia occurs, he has a golden opportunity to draw extra blood for measurements that will help him figure out why the blood sugar fell.

Blood drawn during a fasting attack of hypoglycemia can help the doctor answer the following crucial questions.

When the blood sugar is low, what is the level of insulin in the blood?

When the blood sugar is low, the level of insulin *should* be low also, unless insulin is the cause of the hypoglycemia. In normal people insulin levels rise when the blood sugar rises. The insulin tells fat and muscle tissue to take up the sugar, and tells the liver to store sugar instead of manufacturing and releasing it. When blood sugar levels fall in normal people, their insulin levels also fall, so that the liver will manufacture and release more glucose into the bloodstream, and so that tissues other than the brain won't consume as much glucose. Thus, we know that the insulin level *should be low* when the blood glucose level is low. That is why it is so useful to draw extra blood at the time the blood sugar is low: The doctor can *predict* what levels of insulin and other key components *should* be. By measuring them he can figure out what's wrong.

If the insulin level is appropriately low when the blood sugar is low, the physician knows that the patient is not becoming hypoglycemic because of insulin or other drugs that work through insulin (such as the oral hypoglycemic drugs taken by diabetics). He also knows that the cause of the hypoglycemia is not an insulin-secreting disorder of the pancreas such as tumor or diffuse overgrowth of the islet cells (see Chapters 7 and 8).

On the other hand, if the insulin level is *high* when the blood glucose is low, any of the above problems must be considered as possible culprits. There are also other causes of high insulin levels during fasting hypoglycemia, such as severe infection and erythroblastosis fetalis (Chapters 7 and 8), but in each of these cases, the history and physical examination will already have given good indications of what is going on.

Suppose history and physical examination have given no particular clues to the cause of the low blood sugar, and the doctor has an adult patient with fasting hypoglycemia and a high insulin level. His next question will be, "Where is the insulin coming from?" The laboratory can help him find the answer.

If the insulin level is elevated, what is the source of the insulin?

Persons taking insulin by injection develop anti-insulin antibodies in the bloodstream. Special laboratory tests can detect these antibodies. If the person has just started to take insulin injections, however, the antibodies may be absent. When the excess insulin is coming from a tumor in the pancreas, or from stimulation of the pancreas by a drug, anti-insulin antibodies are generally not found in the bloodstream. The laboratory can still help distinguish among these possibilities, however, by taking advantage of recent progress in understanding how the pancreas normally makes and secretes insulin.

Specialized cells within the pancreas manufacture insulin by first producing a larger molecule named "proinsulin," as shown in Fig. 12. Enzymes within these cells then split off a fragment of the proinsulin molecule known as the "connecting peptide" ("C-peptide" for short). Then, when the cells secrete insulin into the bloodstream, they also secrete the C-peptide fragments along with the insulin. Insulin given by injection, on the other hand, does not contain C-peptide. Therefore, when the doctor finds a high level of insulin in the bloodstream, he can figure out whether it got there by injection or from the pancreas, by also measuring the C-peptide level. If the patient is sneaking insulin injections, or being injected with insulin maliciously by someone else, the C-peptide levels will be low even though the insulin level is high. On the other hand, if the patient has an insulin-producing tumor of the pancreas or is taking a drug, such as chlorpropamide, that stimulates the pancreas to secrete insulin, the C-peptide level will be elevated right along with the insulin level.

Then, you might ask, how can the doctor distinguish between insulin-secreting tumors of the pancreas and the surreptitious use of a drug like chlorpropamide? There are several ways to attack that problem through the laboratory. The doctor could collect the patient's urine and analyze it for chlorpropamide and similar chemicals. He could also measure the blood level of *proinsulin*. When insulin and C-peptide are secreted from a normal pancreas, a very small amount of proinsulin gets secreted along with it. Insulin-secreting tumors, however, usually secrete much more proinsulin. These sophisticated techniques were used to help solve the case of Juan Dominguez.

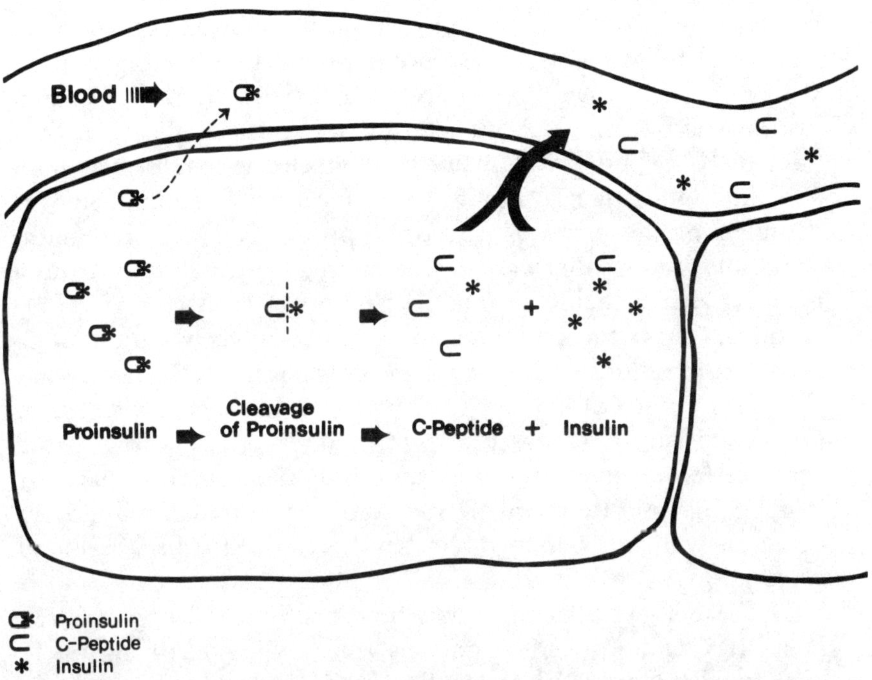

Fig. 12. Schematic diagram of insulin production within the islets of Langerhans. Some proinsulin leaks into the bloodstream, but most of it is split into insulin and C-peptide. C-peptide enters the bloodstream with insulin, as the pancreas secretes them together, in equal amounts.

You may recall from Chapter 2 that because of periods of extreme withdrawal, Juan Dominguez was admitted to a psychiatric ward with the diagnosis of "catatonic schizophrenia." It was found that he had fasting hypoglycemia, and that his symptoms all disappeared when his blood sugar was brought up to normal. Blood taken while his glucose level was very low showed a high insulin level. That meant Juan either was secretly taking insulin shots or some drug that stimulated insulin secretion, or else he had a disorder of the pancreas such as an insulin-producing tumor.

How did we know Juan had a tumor, and wasn't just crazy and taking drugs or shots to make himself sick? After all, he was in the psychiatric ward. We ran laboratory tests that enabled us to distinguish among these possibilities. First, no anti-insulin antibodies were found in his bloodstream. From this information we concluded he probably hadn't been chronically injecting himself with insulin, but we didn't know whether he might have taken just one or two shots about the time of his hospitalization. Second, his C-peptide levels were high when the insulin was high and the blood sugar was low. This meant that the insulin was coming from his pancreas. Third, his proinsulin levels were high, suggesting the insulin was coming from a tumor and not from a normal pancreas being stimulated by a drug. Fourth, tests on his blood and urine turned up no traces of hypoglycemic drugs such as chlorpropamide. Therefore, even though his X-ray didn't show any tumor of his pancreas, we were confident he had one. On this basis we went ahead with surgery. Sure enough, the surgeon found an acorn-sized tumor in the pancreas that was making insulin. Removal of the tumor cured Juan's hypoglycemia, as well as the abnormal behavior resulting from low blood sugar.

The reader can thus appreciate how helpful the laboratory can be in arriving at a specific diagnosis when hypoglycemia is due to high insulin levels. When insulin levels are not inappropriately high, the laboratory can still be of great assistance. It can answer questions such as:

Does the patient have kidney failure?

Since the kidneys filter waste products out of the bloodstream, for disposal in the urine, one finds high levels of waste products in the bloodstream in cases of kidney failure. These are easily detected by inexpensive blood tests in the laboratory. If the waste products are not accumulating in the bloodstream, the kidneys are not sick enough to be the cause of hypoglycemia.

Does the patient have a cancer?

Special X-rays, such as the new computerized body scans, can help answer this question.

Does the patient have severe liver disease?

When the liver is sick, enzymes leak out of the liver into the blood, and can be measured easily. Moreover, the liver has many vital functions besides storing, making, and releasing sugar. It makes proteins necessary for proper blood clotting. A test of the blood's ability to clot will usually be abnormal if a liver disease, such as hepatitis, is severe enough to be the cause of hypoglycemia. In addition, the liver makes a protein called albumin, which is normally present in the blood in large amounts. Liver disease severe enough to cause hypoglycemia will generally also cause a low albumin as well. Easily available lab tests, then, can usually exclude liver disease as the cause of hypoglycemia.

Does the patient have adrenal-gland failure?

If a patient is definitely hypoglycemic after fasting, healthy adrenal glands *should* be secreting cortisol and adrenalin to help bring the blood sugar back up to normal. As mentioned earlier, adrenalin deficiency by itself is not known to be a definite cause of hypoglycemia, but cortisol deficiency is. The specimen of blood drawn during hypoglycemia can be assayed for cortisol. If the cortisol level is elevated, as it should be, adrenal-gland failure cannot be blamed for the hypoglycemia. On the other hand, if it is not elevated during hypoglycemia, adrenal disease is very likely. Further tests can then be done to define whether the adrenal glands are definitely diseased, or whether the pituitary, which is responsible for stimulating the adrenals, is failing.

Does the patient have pituitary-gland failure?

Hypoglycemia will provoke a normal pituitary gland to secrete both growth hormone and the hormone that controls cortisol secretion from the adrenals. By thus measuring growth hormone and cortisol during and shortly after a bout of low blood sugar, the doctor can check on the pituitary and tell whether it is properly secreting those hormones necessary for normal blood sugar.

Does the patient have in the bloodstream all the building blocks necessary to enable the liver to manufacture glucose as needed?

In ketotic hypoglycemia of childhood, kidney failure, cortisol deficiency, and a number of other causes of hypoglycemia, hypoglycemia occurs in part because the liver does not have available in the bloodstream enough building blocks, such as amino acids and glycerol, for gluconeogenesis. These building blocks can be measured in the bloodstream. If adequate levels are found in the blood during hypoglycemia, the doctor can exclude their absence as a cause of the low blood sugar.

The reader will recall from Chapter 6 that three factors are essential for the maintenance of normal blood glucose levels during fasting:

1. A healthy liver,
2. an adequate supply of building blocks for the production of new glucose in the liver (gluconeogenesis), and
3. proper amounts of hormones to regulate the processes of glycogen breakdown and gluconeogenesis.

The preceding paragraphs have explained how each of these essential factors can be checked out through the use of the laboratory. Many other specific tests can also be done to help discover the cause of hypoglycemia, as indicated by the specifics of an individual case. Tests for infection, for the presence of necessary enzymes, and for the availability of alternative fuels, such as ketones, are all available.

One of the more commonly used maneuvers is an injection of glucagon at the time of hypoglycemia. Glucagon will raise the blood sugar in some instances (as when too much insulin is the cause of the low blood sugar), but not in others (such as ketotic hypoglycemia and alcoholic hypoglycemia). In general, glucagon will not raise the blood glucose if liver glycogen stores are depleted, or if the enzymes necessary for glycogen breakdown are absent. This fact has therapeutic as well as diagnostic implications, since glucagon is sometimes used as a treatment for hypoglycemia.

Now that we have reviewed the basics of history, physical examination, and laboratory evaluation, let's apply what we've learned to an actual case of hypoglycemia. Like Watson at the elbow of Sherlock Holmes, see if you can use the knowledge gained from previous chapters to follow the reasoning that solved the mystery.

SOLVING A CASE

Marvin MacDuff, a 46-year-old man, seemed dazed after the auto accident. He couldn't give the police a clear account of why he had run a stop sign and then smashed into a parked vehicle on his way to work that morning. His hand trembled as he fumbled for his driver's license. Because he looked a little uncoordinated, the officers gave him a breath test for alcohol. It was negative. Then as they were completing the accident report, Marvin passed out and started having a convulsion. The police officers weren't sure whether this was just a severe psychological, or hysterical, reaction to his trying circumstances, but thought they'd better play it safe. They drove him with sirens blaring to the emergency room of a nearby hospital. There, blood was drawn for glucose measurement, and intravenous glucose administered, as a matter of routine initial management of unconscious patients.

Marvin came quickly to his senses after receiving the glucose. He was alarmed to find himself in a hospital. He remembered nothing that had happened that morning. When the report of his blood glucose came back at 22 mg/dl, the emergency-room physician decided to admit him to the hospital for immediate evaluation of hypoglycemia. His auto wreck had proved that this was a potentially dangerous condition and immediate investigation seemed in order.

Dr. Holmes was called to figure out why Marvin had low blood sugar. He began by interviewing both Mr. and Mrs. MacDuff.

The MacDuffs claimed Marvin had no previous history of auto accidents or fainting spells or convulsions. They admitted he drank a couple of martinis before dinner most nights after work, but both he and Mrs. MacDuff maintained stoutly that he'd had nothing to drink since before dinner the night before the accident. He took no regular medications. Mrs. MacDuff, on the other hand, was diabetic and took the drug chlorpropamide to lower her blood sugar. Occasionally Marvin got out of bed in the middle of the night to take a sleeping pill to relieve insomnia, but neither he nor his wife recalled anything of the sort the night before the accident.

Dr. Holmes immediately wondered whether Marvin might have accidentally taken one of his wife's pills while getting up groggily in the middle of the night. Or perhaps she was slipping him some without his knowledge. He immediately called the lab and asked the technician to save any remaining serum from the blood tube drawn in the emergency room, so that insulin and drug measurements could be made on it. Unfortunately, the technician had already discarded the specimen.

As questioning of the couple continued, Dr. Holmes learned that their love life had been quite cold lately. Marvin, often out late at night because of work, just hadn't seemed much interested in married life. He was just too tired, Marvin said. Both agreed he'd been kind of depressed and fatigued for the past six or eight months. Mrs. MacDuff had begun to wonder about his fidelity, but confided this to Dr. Holmes only later, in private. These bits of information conjured up all sorts of possibilities in Dr. Holmes's mind, ranging from neurosis, to poisoning, to hormonal deficiencies, to some sort of disease affecting the entire body, such as kidney failure, cancer, or liver disease. Certainly the alcohol intake, often greatly underestimated by patients giving their history, could affect liver function.

Dr. Holmes inquired about Marvin's weight. It had crept up about 10 pounds in the past six months. This would be more consistent with a chronic overabundance of insulin, thought the doctor, as in an insulin-secreting tumor. Lots of alcohol could do the same, though. On the other hand, kidney failure or adrenal disease would be expected to interfere with appetite and lead to weight loss.

A series of questions from Dr. Holmes probed for any possible pattern of hypoglycemic symptoms. There was no history at all of adrenergic symptoms such as tremor, sweating, palpitations, or anxiety. The only symptom suggesting possible brain malfunction, apart from the day of the accident, was a headache that had been present most mornings for the past month. Marvin would often awaken tired, with a dull aching of the entire head that would subside after breakfast. Perhaps Mr. MacDuff was becoming hypoglycemic overnight in his sleep, thought the doctor, or maybe this was just a hangover, or the effects of high blood pressure.

Despite detailed questioning, Dr. Holmes turned up no further clues from Mr. MacDuff's history. The next step was to examine him.

Marvin's blood pressure turned out to be perfectly normal—if anything a bit on the low side, at 110/70. This made high blood pressure untenable as an explanation for the morning headache. Except for mild overweight and slight softening of the testicles, Mr. MacDuff's physical examination was perfectly normal.

Dr. Holmes decided next to find out whether Mr. MacDuff

would become hypoglycemic while fasting in the hospital under direct observation. That way he could be sure that Marvin wasn't intentionally taking something to reduce his own blood glucose. In the controlled conditions of the hospital, Dr. Holmes could also exclude the possibility of poisoning. If Marvin's blood sugar dropped abnormally low while fasting in the hospital, under observation, off all drugs and alcohol, it would mean there was something definitely wrong with Marvin's metabolism. Dr. Holmes knew that normal men do not drop their plasma glucose below 55 mg/dl in a 72-hour fast.

Dr. Holmes told Marvin he was ordering a nurse's aide to be in attendance with him at all times, so that if symptoms occurred they would be noticed before progressing to unconsciousness. A blood sugar was to be ordered right away if Marvin started to act strangely or experienced any symptoms of hypoglycemia. Extra blood was also to be drawn for measurement of insulin if the blood sugar turned out to be definitely low. The fast began after breakfast on Sunday morning.

Monday morning, after 24 hours without food, Mr. MacDuff's plasma glucose was 55 mg/dl, and he felt perfectly well. He didn't even have a headache that morning. Dr. Holmes began to wonder whether Marvin really had spontaneous hypoglycemia after all. He decided to prolong the fast.

By 6:00 P.M. Monday night, the plasma glucose was 51 mg/dl, but apart from fatigue and mild hunger, Marvin felt well. His brain was functioning normally, and he had no feelings of shakiness or anxiety. He was not sweating, and his heart rate was a leisurely 60 beats per minute. Not satisfied that 51 mg/dl was definitely low, Dr. Holmes decided to continue the fast.

Tuesday morning Marvin awoke feeling tired, with a headache. His plasma glucose was 42 mg/dl. "Aha," thought Holmes, "now we really have something here! If we can just drive his blood sugar a little farther down, we'll know he has hypoglycemia and that his insulin level *should* be low. If the insulin level is high, while the blood sugar is low, we'll focus our search on those causes of hypoglycemia that act through insulin. On the other hand, if the insulin level is low, all those causes can be eliminated from consideration."

Dr. Holmes called the laboratory and asked for a technician who drew blood to come to the bedside. Then Dr. Holmes invited the technician to join him and Marvin for a stroll. They walked down the hall to the stairwell, then up one flight. Then back down a flight. Then up and down four more times. Mr. MacDuff began feeling weak and shaky. He looked pale, and was perspiring lightly. When Holmes asked him his telephone number, he couldn't remember it. Dr. Holmes took hold of his wrist and found the pulse racing at 120 beats per minute. He had the laboratory technician draw several tubes of blood from Marvin's arm and requested that the blood glucose measurements be run immediately and the rest of the blood saved.

Dr. Holmes then reached in his black bag and produced a bottle of Lucozade, a popular British soft drink with a high glucose content, and gave it to the weak and befuddled Mr. MacDuff. Within five minutes of drinking it, Mr. MacDuff felt better, and could recite his telephone number quickly and easily. Dr. Holmes called the lab and asked the technician to return promptly and draw more blood, for glucose and cortisol and growth-hormone measurements.

The plasma glucose drawn in the stairwell during symptoms was 31 mg/dl. Twenty minutes later, when he was feeling better after the sugar intake, Mr. MacDuff's glucose level was up to 68 mg/dl.

Holmes concluded that MacDuff did indeed have hypoglycemia, that it occurred in the fasting state, and that it was apparently not due to any drug or alcohol he had been taking.

The extra blood taken when MacDuff's blood sugar was low, at 31 mg/dl, was sent first for insulin measurement. The insulin level turned out to be low. This excluded an insulin-secreting tumor, and was evidence that Marvin hadn't been secretly taking insulin, or getting drugs, like his wife's chlorpropamide, that could lower the blood sugar by stimulating the pancreas to secrete insulin. Since there was no excess of insulin, there must be either a deficiency of anti-insulin hormones, or something wrong with the liver, or a lack of enzymes or building blocks necessary for glucose production in the liver. The easiest of these possibilities to exclude was a sick liver. Blood tests showed no excess amounts of the enzymes that would leak into the bloodstream from a damaged liver, and no deficiency of albumin or blood-clotting factors that the liver produces. Severe liver disease was ruled out. The anti-insulin hormones took a little longer to measure.

Within a week, first the cortisol and then the growth-hormone measurements became available. They were both abnormally low for someone with a definitely low blood sugar. Since growth hormone comes from the pituitary gland, and cortisol comes from the adrenals, which are controlled by the pituitary, the lack of both these hormones pointed directly to Mr. MacDuff's pituitary gland as the cause of hypoglycemia. Dr. Holmes had already suspected the pituitary gland, since it also controls the testicles, which produce testosterone, the hormone that gives men a normal sex drive. Dr. Holmes had noticed the history of a lessening love life, plus softening of the testicles on physical examination. He had therefore already ordered a test for the blood level of testosterone, and it too was abnormally low.

Fatigue and weight gain were the other symptoms possibly attributable to a pituitary-gland problem, since the thyroid gland, which depends on the pituitary for stimulation, makes a hormone necessary for normal zest and energy expenditure. MacDuff's thyroid-hormone level was also lower than normal. All of these hormones—growth hormone, thyroid hormone, testosterone, and cortisol—can be given by mouth or by injection, so treatment by replacing these missing hormones was available. In fact, when the other hormones are replaced, growth hormone need not be replaced in an adult such as Mr. MacDuff. Before proceeding with hormone replacement, however, Dr. Holmes wanted to answer a final, crucial question: *Why* was Marvin MacDuff's pituitary gland not functioning normally?

Since Marvin's pituitary gland was not functioning normally, there had to be something wrong with it. Intelligent treatment depended on discovering what was wrong so that appropriate treatment could be given. Dr. Holmes ordered a specialized X-ray of the pituitary gland, using one of the very newest computerized scanners that can see small tumors within the pituitary.

The X-ray showed an abnormal mass within the pituitary gland, smashing the normal pituitary tissue against the walls of its bony socket. Since further enlargement of a pituitary tumor can endanger nearby vital structures, such as the nerves to the eyes, Dr. Holmes asked Mr. MacDuff to consent to an operation on his pituitary gland.

Mr. MacDuff objected. He had read somewhere that if one has hypoglycemia, all you need is vitamin supplements and a special low-carbohydrate, high-protein diet taken in six meals per day. He wanted to try that approach first. Dr. Holmes said no, Marvin didn't need treatment for a disease he didn't have. If his hypoglycemia had been of the reactive type, which occurs after meals in people who have had stomach surgery for ulcers, that sort of diet would make sense. But Marvin's disease was an abnormal growth within the pituitary, interfering with proper function of the rest of the gland. He needed treatment for the disease that was causing his hypoglycemia.

Marvin finally consented to the operation. With Marvin under general anesthesia, a neurosurgeon made an incision above the gums inside Marvin's upper lip, removed some bone, and opened a passageway up through the nose and sinuses to the bony cavity of the pituitary gland. The surgeon peeled away this bone, exposing the pituitary to view. The abnormal growth turned out to be a fluid-filled cyst. The neurosurgeon removed the cyst completely, and left the rest of the pituitary gland intact.

After the operation Marvin healed, and noted a gradual return of his normal energy, sex drive, and sense of well-being. The pituitary, no longer compressed within its bony socket, began to function normally once more. His blood hormone levels of testosterone, growth hormone, cortisol, and thyroid hormone all returned to normal, without the need for pills or injections for replacement. Marvin was cured. His blood sugar level remained normal.

Hypoglycemia had not been Marvin's disease; it was a manifestation of his disease. His disease was pituitary-gland failure caused by a benign cyst. Appropriate treatment of the disease relieved the manifestations of the disease, including fatigue, lack of sex drive, weight gain, and hypoglycemia. Before Marvin's disease could be intelligently treated, the specific cause of his hypoglycemia had to be diagnosed, by the brilliant Dr. Holmes. When you understand what hypoglycemia is all about, it is really rather elementary. Don't you think so, Watson?

SUMMARY

To summarize the main points of this chapter:

1. Before embarking on a search for the specific cause of someone's hypoglycemia, first make sure that person really does have abnormally low blood sugar.

2. A qualified physician is needed to help define the cause of any individual case of hypoglycemia.
3. The medical history provides important clues, especially regarding the timing of symptoms in relation to meals, exercise, and fasting.
4. Other information, such as drugs and alcohol usage, pregnancy, and other diseases and symptoms, is also helpful.
5. Physical examination, though especially important in children, is seldom sufficient to give a specific diagnosis. Laboratory tests are needed.
6. Judicious use of the laboratory will usually permit the physician to reach a definite diagnosis in cases of authentic hypoglycemia.

Specific diagnosis leads directly to appropriate treatment, the subject of our next chapter.

10

How Should Hypoglycemia Be Treated and Prevented?

The title of this chapter is a trick question. As you know from reading the first nine chapters of this book, hypoglycemia is not a single disease. It is a manifestation of some underlying disease or problem. The long-term treatment depends on what that problem is. In the short term, however, it is often necessary to raise the blood sugar immediately, even before a more specific diagnosis of the problem has been made. In this chapter we shall first consider the immediate, short-term correction of hypoglycemia, and then the long-term treatment of underlying causes. Prevention of hypoglycemia flows naturally from correction of its underlying causes.

THE IMMEDIATE TREATMENT OF LOW BLOOD SUGAR

In theory, one could raise the blood glucose level promptly either by speeding up the input of glucose into the bloodstream or by cutting off its outflow. In practice, because the brain requires a continuing supply of glucose from the bloodstream, cutting off glucose outflow is not a realistic choice When your blood sugar is too low, you need an immediate surge in glucose input.

GLUCOSE BY VEIN

The quickest way to put glucose into the circulation is through a needle. The intravenous administration of 25 grams of glucose will raise anyone's blood sugar. Hypoglycemic symptoms will disappear promptly, unless prolonged hypoglycemia has caused lasting damage.

Sterile vials containing 25 grams of glucose in 50 milliliters (about 1½ ounces) of water are widely available in hospitals and doctor's offices. They are used for intravenous injection in emergency situations, such as coma or convulsions caused by hypoglycemia. When symptoms are not so severe, the intravenous route of glucose administration is not usually necessary, and the sugar can be given by mouth instead.

GLUCOSE BY MOUTH

When you eat glucose, your stomach and intestines absorb it promptly into your bloodstream. Many foods contain glucose in quickly absorbable form. Oranges, orange juice, other fruits and their juices, sugar cubes, Life-Savers, and soda pop are favorite "standby" remedies for low blood sugar, but countless other foods are perfectly adequate as well. The key ingredient is rapidly absorbable carbohydrate. Diet soda will *not* serve, for example, because it contains non-sugar sweeteners instead of glucose.

Companies have begun to manufacture and market tablets of dextrose (glucose) specifically for the immediate treatment of hypoglycemia, but these products offer no real advantage over candy or some other quickly absorbable sugar source. Their advertisers may contend that conventional sugar is made of sucrose, which has to be broken down to glucose before you can absorb it, whereas their product consists of glucose already in the absorbable form. In fact, however, your enzymes split sucrose so rapidly into its component glucose molecules that it serves the purpose of promptly raising the blood glucose perfectly well.

If a person can eat, he can raise the blood sugar in a hurry by consuming some sugary or starchy food. But when someone cannot eat, as when in coma from hypoglycemia, glucose by vein is the best remedy, provided the necessary materials are available. The necessary materials include someone who knows how to give an intravenous injection. If the requisite skill and materials are not available, glucagon provides another option.

GLUCAGON BY INJECTION

Glucagon is the anti-insulin hormone that raises blood glucose mainly by promoting glycogen breakdown. With little or no training, almost anyone can give an injection of glucagon into the muscle of someone unconscious from hypoglycemia. The muscles of the thigh are an easy target, though many people use the shoulder muscle or the buttocks instead. Once delivered into the muscle, glucagon passes into the bloodstream and raises the blood sugar within 15 or 20 minutes.

Since glucagon works primarily through the liberation of glucose stored as glycogen, it is especially effective in situations in which the liver contains plenty of glycogen. An overdose of insulin is a good example of this kind of situation. On the other hand, glucagon does not work well in cases of hypoglycemia characterized by the absence of liver glycogen. Examples of hypoglycemia in which the liver lacks glycogen include (1) severe starvation, (2) ketotic hypoglycemia of childhood, and (3) alcoholic hypoglycemia in the fasting state, as occurred with Sherry Tippler in Chapter 6. Glucagon would not help in such cases.

Many families of diabetic patients keep glucagon handy in the refrigerator. When a diabetic patient's blood glucose drops too low because of too much insulin and exercise or not enough food, the hypoglycemia can generally be corrected by taking glucose by mouth. If matters have progressed to coma, however, the family usually cannot get the patient to swallow anything. By giving the patient an injection of glucagon they can raise his blood sugar within 15 or 20 minutes—probably sooner than they could get him to a hospital emergency room. Families may use the same needle and syringe for the glucagon as the patient uses for insulin.

Once glucose or glucagon has relieved the immediate crisis, the next order of business is to determine *why* the blood sugar fell and to take steps to ensure that it won't happen again. In the previous chapter we discussed how to find out why the blood sugar fell. Let's now cover what to do about it once a specific diagnosis has been made.

THE LONG-TERM TREATMENT AND PREVENTION OF HYPOGLYCEMIA

The treatment of any particular case of hypoglycemia depends on its cause. The situation is similar to anemia. A blood transfusion will temporarily correct anemia (low blood hemoglobin level) in anyone. The long-term cure, however, depends on why the blood hemoglobin is low. It could be anything from an operation to remove a bleeding tumor to injections of vitamin B_{12}. So it is also for low blood sugar. Once the underlying cause has been defined, appropriate therapy becomes obvious.

We shall consider the therapies and preventions available for some of the most interesting and most common causes of hypoglycemia. As you will see, the rational treatment of hypoglycemia simply exploits what is known about human glucose metabolism, as explained in the preceding chapters. The more that medical scientists learn about what controls blood sugar, the more avenues for preventing and relieving hypoglycemia become available.

HYPOGLYCEMIA IN NEWBORNS

In addition to general measures such as feeding newborn babies promptly and frequently, specific measures can correct many causes of hypoglycemia in this age group. As discussed in Chapter 8, erythroblastosis fetalis is becoming rare as doctors now prevent Rh-negative mothers from becoming sensitized to the Rh-positive blood of their offspring.

Modern obstetrical care can also reduce prematurity, an important cause of hypoglycemia in newborns. For example, there used to be some guesswork in trying to time the delivery when a woman needed a Cesarean section or induction of labor by drugs. Now, by using a technique known as amniocentesis, doctors can determine prior to birth whether a baby is still premature. In this technique the doctor inserts a needle into the uterus to obtain a sample of the amniotic fluid surrounding the fetus. By analyzing the chemical composition of the fluid, the doctor can estimate the degree of physical maturity of the unborn baby. Then, if the baby is still immature, Cesarean section or the induction of labor can be postponed.

Infants of diabetic mothers have been particularly prone to hypoglycemia, because the huge amount of glucose coming across the placenta from the mother stimulates too much insulin secretion in the baby. This problem is now becoming less frequent as doctors and diabetic patients control the mother's blood sugar more carefully before childbirth. New devices, such as portable pumps for giving insulin in a precisely controlled manner, and devices for measuring one's own blood sugar, make it possible for the pregnant diabetic woman to keep her blood sugar in the normal range much better now than ever before. With the mother's blood glucose controlled in the near-normal range, the fetus is not exposed to so much sugar. Consequently, its pancreas is less stimulated to produce insulin, and after delivery there is less of a downward overshoot of the blood glucose. This is a good example of how medical research, by discovering the specific mechanisms causing hypoglycemia, paves the way for prevention.

HYPOGLYCEMIA IN CHILDREN

Diffuse overgrowth of the islet cells produces hypoglycemia that can be difficult and complex to treat. Those cases in which the amino acid leucine triggers the excessive insulin release ("leucine sensitivity"—see Chapter 8) may benefit from dietary restriction. Leucine is so widespread in foods, however, that its total elimination from the diet is not practical. Diet may help, but by itself seldom suffices to prevent hypoglycemia in these children. Since unrelenting insulin secretion leads to prolonged and severe hypoglycemia, with resulting brain damage, effective treatment is essential. Doctors therefore resort to additional measures, such as drugs and surgery.

The first operation usually done in cases of diffuse islet-cell overgrowth is the removal of about 80% of the pancreas. This procedure carries a mortality rate (risk of death) of about 10% or more, but often succeeds in relieving the hypoglycemia. In some cases, the entire pancreas must be removed before the blood sugar can be controlled.

In addition to the risk of death, removal of the pancreas can cause diabetes, as well as a lack of digestive enzymes with consequent poor absorption of food and malnutrition. We try, therefore, to avoid this operation when possible, especially since some of these patients seem to get better gradually on their own. Other measures, such as drugs, may help support the glucose level in the normal range and allow us to postpone surgery.

The drug most often used to treat diffuse islet-cell overgrowth is called diazoxide. Used in combination with a closely related drug, chlorothiazide, it partially blocks insulin secretion from the pancreas. A newly discovered hormone, somatostatin, also blocks the secretion of insulin. As medical research continues, this hormone may come to play a greater part in the treatment of diffuse islet-cell overgrowth. Indeed, scientists theorize that a deficiency of somatostatin may cause the overgrowth of insulin-producing cells in some of these cases.

Other measures used to support the level of blood sugar in cases of islet-cell overgrowth include administration of the anti-insulin hormones cortisol and glucagon. Cortisol is usually given by mouth in the form of hydrocortisone. It has severe side effects if given in large doses for a long time. Glucagon is given by injection in a long-acting form known as zinc glucagon.

When the cause of hypoglycemia is a *missing or defective enzyme* necessary for glucose production, administration of anti-insulin hormones such as glucagon may not help. These patients already have the necessary hormones; they lack the cellular machinery (enzymes) to respond to the hormones. We have no way to repair enzymes at the present time. All we can do is bypass their function, usually by providing glucose orally.

Frequent meals provide a fairly steady flow of glucose into the bloodstream of these patients during the day. At night, a thin tube slipped through the nose and down the throat into the stomach provides a means of continuing glucose input. Glucose-containing liquid formula is pumped slowly down the tube throughout the night. Breakfast is taken before the tube is removed, to assure an uninterrupted supply of carbohydrate. Although cumbersome, this logical treatment greatly benefits patients with hypoglycemia caused by some types of inherited enzyme defects.

Other enzyme problems cause severe hypoglycemia after intake of certain non-glucose sugars. For example, fructose or galactose can cause hypoglycemia and other chemical abnormalities, sometimes severe enough to cause death, in persons with hereditary fructose intolerance or galactosemia. Treatment consists of modifying the diet to exclude the offending substances.

Ketotic hypoglycemia of childhood is also treated primarily through diet. You will recall that these children cannot maintain the new production of glucose (gluconeogenesis) between meals because of their low blood levels of the necessary building blocks. A *high*-carbohydrate diet taken in four or more feedings per day, including a large bedtime snack, prevents the hypoglycemia. The copious carbohydrates provide plenty of sugar for production of glycogen, which then supplies glucose between meals.

Note that the high carbohydrate content of this diet is opposite the current fad diets for hypoglycemia, which imitate the dietary therapy of reactive hypoglycemia following ulcer surgery.

Hydrocortisone, given at bedtime, also prevents overnight fasting hypoglycemia in these children. It raises the blood levels of alanine, thus permitting gluconeogenesis to proceed normally. The potential side effects of hydrocortisone, however, make it a choice of last resort. Most patients manage well with diet alone.

HYPOGLYCEMIA FROM CAUSES COMMON TO ADULTS AND CHILDREN

Lack of anti-insulin hormones is treated simply by replacing the missing hormones. Some can be given by mouth; others require injection. Such treatment is so logical that it underscores the absurdity of recommending a high-protein, low-carbohydrate diet for all cases of hypoglycemia. The treatment depends on the disease.

Drugs, poisonings, alcohol, ackee fruit, and oral glucose tolerance tests—avoidance of these substances will obviously prevent the hypoglycemia they cause. Merely reducing the dosage of a drug often eliminates the side effect of hypoglycemia. People who find abstinence from alcohol an unacceptable alternative can prevent their blood sugar from falling by continuing to eat during and after alcohol intake. Though they may become fat and drunk, at least they do so with a normal blood glucose level.

Kidney failure, if complete and permanent, is best treated by kidney transplant when a suitable donor is available. The "artificial kidney machines," which successfully prolong the lives of thousands of people, do not prevent the hypoglycemia of kidney failure. Frequent feedings of carbohydrate-rich food, including a snack in the middle of the night, help lessen hypoglycemia in these patients.

Severe heart disease and *severe, widespread infection* are treated by drugs or surgery, or both, depending on the exact nature of the problem. Curing the heart disease or the infection will also correct the hypoglycemia they cause.

The treatment of *severe liver disease* remains primitive. We remove offending substances, try to maintain ideal nutrition, and hope the liver will heal. Certain types of liver disease are treated with hydrocortisone or related drugs, a side effect of which can be the elevation of blood glucose levels.

Insulinomas should be removed surgically when possible, as in the case of Juan Dominguez (Chapter 7). Approximately 80% of insulinomas are solitary and benign (i.e., not cancerous). The challenge is to find the tumor and take it out. They can be hard to find. X-rays sometimes help locate the tumor before surgery, but often, as in Juan's case, the surgeon opens the abdomen without knowing exactly where the tumor lurks. The surgeon explores the pancreas feeling for a lump that will prove to be the tumor. If he or she cannot find such a lump, the surgeon may remove a portion of the pancreas in hopes that the tumor will be within the part removed.

About 10% of insulinomas are multiple, but not malignant. That is, there are several of them but they're not spreading. Removal of part of the pancreas may help, but seldom cures, these cases. The other 10% of insulinomas are cancerous, spreading within the pancreas and to the liver. Once such a tumor has spread to the liver, surgical cure is virtually impossible. In these cases, as in diffuse islet-cell overgrowth and benign insulinomas that elude complete removal, drugs help curtail the secretion of insulin.

Diazoxide and chlorothiazide inhibit insulin secretion and are the most widely used drugs for treatment of insulinoma. Other drugs that also lessen the secretion of insulin include phenytoin and propranolol. These may be used in addition to diazoxide. When a malignant islet-cell tumor continues to spread and to secrete too much insulin, the doctor may turn to a more toxic type of drug that actually destroys the insulin-producing cells. These drugs should be used only by experts, and only in proved cases of insulin overproduction caused by tumor or overgrowth of the islet cells.

HYPOGLYCEMIA IN ADULTS

The conditions discussed above occur in adults as well as children, whereas those that follow occur almost exclusively in adults. As in children, the long-term treatment of hypoglycemia in adults would ideally consist of correcting the underlying problem. When this is not possible, an indirect approach, based on an understanding of glucose metabolism and the specific disorder involved, may relieve the hypoglycemia.

Early pregnancy is a cause of fasting hypoglycemia, and the avoidance of prolonged fasting in this "delicate condition" prevents the blood sugar from falling too low. The consumption of frequent meals is often easier said than done, however, since many women suffer intense nausea during the first few months of pregnancy.

Reactive hypoglycemia following ulcer surgery may be treated by further surgery, by diet, or by both. The ulcer surgery that causes hypoglycemia does so by creating an enlarged, wide-open exit pathway from the stomach to the small intestine. This allows very rapid evacuation of the stomach after eating. Repeat surgery to reduce the size of the exit from the stomach can help slow the emptying process. So can surgery that reverses the direction of a segment of small intestine next to the stomach exit. The propulsive contractions of the reversed segment tend to push food back toward the stomach. Both operations reduce the rapidity of stomach emptying. Consequently, blood sugar rises less rapidly after a meal, less insulin is secreted, and the rebound drop in blood sugar due to the insulin is less precipitate. Modifications of diet also aim to reduce insulin secretion by slowing the surge of sugar into the bloodstream.

The most common treatment of reactive hypoglycemia following ulcer surgery is a diet restricted in carbohydrate, especially in refined sugar, consumed in frequent, small meals. Since fructose does not stimulate insulin secretion, it can substitute for glucose in the diet to provide both sweet taste and balanced nutrition without provoking rebound hypoglycemia. A similar strategy is involved in the use of a high-fiber diet, which slows carbohydrate absorption, and also in the use of drugs that slow the emptying of the stomach.

Some recently popularized substances inhibit the enzymes that break sucrose and starch down into individual glucose molecules. While these substances slow the absorption of glucose, they cause cramps and gas in many people, because the carbohydrate that is not absorbed into the bloodstream stays in the intestines. There the bacteria attack it, utilize it for fuel, and make gas as a byproduct. Most people find this approach unacceptable, though it has been tried in cases of reactive hypoglycemia both with and without prior ulcer surgery.

Hypoglycemia caused by rapid stomach emptying in the absence of ulcer surgery is a controversial area. Proof that the spontaneous symptoms in these patients are really accompanied by low blood glucose is lacking in most reports. Nevertheless, some people diagnosed merely by glucose tolerance testing have reported improvement following treatment with propantheline, which slows the contractions that empty the stomach. This treatment, like the diet for hypoglycemia patients whose stomachs have lost their holding action because of surgery, has also been prescribed to many persons diagnosed as having idiopathic reactive hypoglycemia.

Idiopathic reactive hypoglycemia has no intelligent, reliable treatment because:

1. by definition, we don't know what causes it, and
2. scientific literature on the subject has been muddled by two problems:
   a. Most alleged cases have been diagnosed by oral glucose tolerance testing, not by the finding of abnormal blood sugar levels during daily symptoms.
   b. Well-designed studies, with controls to correct for the "placebo effect" of psychological suggestion which accompanies any therapy, are lacking.

Thus, though the successful treatment of a number of cases has been reported in medical journals, a critical appraisal of those reports leads to the conclusion that we really don't know whether most of those people really had anything wrong with their glucose metabolism in the first place, nor whether the treatment given provided any more benefit than sugar pills would have. I hope that no readers of this book will pursue such remedies before it has been established that their everyday symptoms are due to abnormally low blood sugar, and that the *known* causes of hypoglycemia have been looked for and excluded. With these reservations in mind, let me share with you some of the recently advocated remedies.

First and foremost, the diet appropriate for reactive hypoglycemia after ulcer surgery has been promoted as the remedy for all reactive hypoglycemia. Low in carbohydrates, and therefore high in protein (and fat, in most cases), taken in frequent small feedings, often with various vitamin supplementations, this diet has been the mainstay of popular treatment for hypoglycemia. As often as not it has been applied to people who have never been properly proved to have hypoglycemia at all. Some obese persons have lost weight on the diet, and have thereby benefited, though a more balanced diet would have been preferable. Many versions of the diet are high in animal fat, a problem some people circumvent by choosing vegetable sources of protein, such as beans.

An unfounded but widely applied treatment for idiopathic hypoglycemia has been so-called ACE or "adrenal cortical extract." This treatment originated from the fact that adrenal-gland failure (such as in the case of Enrique Engelhardt, Chapter 1) can cause hypoglycemia. In fact, adrenal insufficiency is a very rare cause of hypoglycemia, and ACE is not an adequate remedy for it. An accurate, authoritative summary of the use of ACE for reactive hypoglycemia was published jointly in 1973 by the American Diabetes Association, the Endocrine Society, and the American Medical Association:

> Adrenal insufficiency is the inability of the adrenal gland to respond to certain bodily needs, especially in times of stress. The diagnosis of this condition requires sophisticated measurements of adrenal hormones in blood or urine. Although hypoglycemia can be one symptom of adrenal insufficiency, adrenal insufficiency, itself an uncommon condition, is a *rare* cause of hypoglycemia. The treatment of adrenal insufficiency has been clarified and made routine by the discovery of cortisone and similar hormones more than 25 years ago. Before this the treatment of adrenal insufficiency was difficult and inadequate. One of the earliest substances tested was adrenal cortical extract, a preparation of beef or pork adrenal glands. This material proved to be relatively useless because the necessary adrenal hormones are present only in minimal amounts. Since highly purified individual adrenal hormones are now available to take by mouth, adrenal cortical extract is of historical interest only, and there is no known medical use for it. In fact, the few drug companies still manufacturing this preparation do not list treatment of hypoglycemia as one of its uses. Thus it should be stressed that administration of

adrenal cortical extract is not an appropriate treatment for any cause of hypoglycemia.[1]

Propantheline, which slows stomach emptying, has been tried in many people diagnosed as having idiopathic reactive hypoglycemia, and some of them have felt better. Propantheline does help prevent hypoglycemia during an oral glucose tolerance test, but we don't know whether it changes blood sugar levels in everyday life, nor whether the blood sugar of most of the people so treated was really responsible for their symptoms.

Oral hypoglycemic medications are used in the treatment of mild diabetes mellitus. You may recall their use in the story of Stella Sharp, in Chapter 5. On the unsubstantiated theory that hypoglycemia is an early stage of diabetes mellitus, she took chlorpropamide. Stella felt worse, but some people treated in this manner have felt better, including some with prior ulcer surgery. Unfortunately, like other drug therapies for reactive hypoglycemia, this approach is not substantiated by any well-designed studies. Most people with mild diabetes mellitus are overweight; they do not need a drug, like chlorpropamide, that promotes further weight gain. They need to lose weight by cutting down on calories and exercising more. Most of them will feel better if they do so.

Propranolol is another drug reported to help in the treatment of hypoglycemia. Once again, the published reports do not make it clear that hypoglycemia actually caused the symptoms in the first place. Propranolol blocks many actions of adrenalin, so it would be expected to prevent and relieve adrenergic symptoms, even in the absence of hypoglycemia. If a person really had hypoglycemia, propranolol would be an illogical choice since it would mask the warning symptoms and impair the corrective mechanisms that raise blood glucose back to normal. On the other hand, in some cases of symptoms *without* hypoglycemia ("nonhypoglycemia"), propranolol can be quite useful.

NONHYPOGLYCEMIA

How should those thousands of people be treated who have symptoms that are popularly attributed to hypoglycemia, but that in fact are *not* due to low blood sugar?

[1] M. B. Davidson, Chairman, Ad Hoc Committee on Hypoglycemia, *Annals of Internal Medicine* 78 (1973), 301.

Obviously, there is no single, simple answer to that question. The proper treatment depends on what is causing the symptoms in each individual case.

Some such people have apparently felt better after applying the remedies listed above, though cause and effect remain obscure. Some people with adrenergic symptoms such as shakiness and rapid heartbeat benefit from an adrenalin-blocking drug such as propranolol. Those with thyroid disease should improve as that problem is corrected. Those with anxiety or depression may benefit from counseling, medication, a new job, or a vacation. Those with intolerance to certain foods may feel better if they avoid those foods. Those who are obese may respond to weight reduction. Let us not suppose, however, that by incorrectly labeling these people as having hypoglycemia we are in any way promoting their health. The remedies listed above can be tried without pretending that the blood sugar is involved. Moreover, if there is comfort in being told that something specific is wrong, such reassurance can be honestly offered without inventing a fiction about blood glucose.

SUMMARY

To summarize the treatment of hypoglycemia:

1. Hypoglycemia requires immediate correction. Food intake, glucose injection, and in some instances glucagon injection will raise the blood sugar promptly.
2. The long-term prevention and treatment of hypoglycemia depend on what is causing it.
3. Treatment of the underlying cause will relieve or prevent the hypoglycemia.
4. When the underlying cause cannot be cured, as in inherited enzyme deficiencies, the application of scientific knowledge about glucose metabolism often provides a means to keep the blood sugar normal.
5. Don't embark on long-term treatment for hypoglycemia until you have evidence that low blood sugar is really the cause of your symptoms.

Now let's go on to other guidelines for persons suspected of having hypoglycemia.

11

Advice for Persons Suspected of Having Hypoglycemia

Many thousands of people have been told that they have hypoglycemia. Thousands of others suspect they *might* have it. This entire book aims to inform and help such people. The present chapter summarizes what they should and shouldn't *do* about their suspected case of low blood sugar.

1. Read Chapters 1 through 4. After reading the first four chapters of this book, you should understand that hypoglycemia can manifest itself through a great variety of symptoms. Two people with hypoglycemia might experience entirely different symptoms, though in any one person the symptoms tend to be repetitive from one episode of low blood sugar to the next.

You should also understand that the symptoms of hypoglycemia are not diagnostic. They are not specific for hypoglycemia. Since many other conditions can cause similar symptoms, you cannot be sure you have hypoglycemia until your blood sugar has been measured during symptoms and found to be abnormally low. Moreover, intake of sugar should promptly relieve your symptoms if they are due to hypoglycemia. If after reading Chapters 1 through 4 you feel that your symptoms could be due to low blood sugar, you should see your doctor.

2. Discuss your concerns with your doctor. At this point you do not need a specialist in blood glucose metabolism. You need a sympathetic, intelligent, well-trained physician to consider your symptoms. Your own family doctor would be ideal, since presumably he already knows you and your medical background, and you have confidence in his care and skill. While giving consideration to the possibility of hypoglycemia, he may think of other conditions that could be contributing to your symptoms. For example, having taken care of your mother's overactive thyroid, he would be in a position to suspect a similar problem when you come in with shakiness, rapid heartbeat, and profuse perspiration. He may thus be able to pinpoint your problem without your even having to pay for measurement of your blood sugar. But if he does think that hypoglycemia is a real possibility, the next step is to measure your blood glucose during the symptoms that make you and your doctor suspect it may be subnormal.

3. Obtain accurate measurement of your blood sugar during symptoms. As explained in Chapter 4, this may require ingenuity. It is worth the effort, however, to be certain that your day-to-day symptoms are really linked to the level of your blood glucose. Your physician can put you in contact with a laboratory that will measure your blood glucose. I strongly recommend that this be done in a professional, licensed laboratory experienced in measuring blood glucose. Since we are basing the entire decision of whether to pursue the diagnosis of hypoglycemia on the measurement of your blood sugar during symptoms, that measurement must be reliable.

New devices have recently become available for the lay person to use in measuring his or her own blood glucose at home. They are extremely useful in the treatment of *high* blood sugar (diabetes mellitus). If they could be relied upon to give values consistently *accurate* to within 2% or 3% of the actual blood glucose value, they could be used to figure out whether someone has hypoglycemia. Unfortunately, their accuracy is more in the range of plus or minus 10% to 15%, *after* one has been trained and certified in their use.

In managing patients with diabetes, I have seen repeated instances of 50% to 100% error in the measurement of blood glucose with these devices. Therefore, I always insist that diabetics using them *verify* the accuracy of their technique by measuring their blood sugar at the same time a chemistry laboratory does, on several occasions, until they can repeatedly show that they get a value within 10% to 15% of the chemistry laboratory. This requires several trips to the laboratory. It is not worth the bother and expense to go through all this training and certification just to use the device for measurement of blood glucose at home on six or seven occasions. Moreover, since even in trained hands their accuracy is only plus or minus 10% to 15%, these devices are not accurate enough to sort out the significance of readings in the borderline range of blood sugars between 40 and 60 mg/dl. It is simpler and more reliable just to use the chemistry laboratory for measurement of your blood glucose during symptoms.

On the other hand, if you have a neighbor or family member with diabetes who has one of these devices, and who is experienced in its use, and who has proved by simultaneous chemistry-lab determinations that his or her technique is accurate within 10%, you might be able to *exclude* hypoglycemia as a cause of your symptoms with reasonable confidence. For example, if your blood sugar is measured at 100 to 120 mg/dl during symptoms, by someone with verified accuracy in the usage of one of these devices, you can be reasonably reassured that your blood sugar is not below 60 mg/dl, and therefore not even in the borderline "gray zone."

The above paragraphs contain so many cautions and qualifiers that I suggest that instead you deal directly with a professional chemistry laboratory, so that you can rely on the results. Ideally, you would visit the lab on several occasions during symptoms, to be sure that what you are experiencing is really due to low blood sugar.

Some of your symptoms may be due to hypoglycemia, and others not. Therefore it is helpful to keep a log of your symptoms at the times your blood sugar is drawn, so that later you can sit down with your doctor and compare specific symptoms to their corresponding blood glucose values. In this way you can focus in on which, if any, of your symptoms arise from low blood sugar. Those symptoms that are not hypoglycemic in nature deserve evaluation too. Just because some of your symptoms are not due to hypoglycemia doesn't mean they should be dismissed. Thus, the first step is to sort out which symptoms in daily living are accompanied by abnormally low blood sugar levels.

Once you have documented that your blood sugar during symptoms is definitely low, the next step is to find out *why* it is low.

4. Press for a specific diagnosis. At this point it would be premature to prescribe a long-term treatment for your hypoglycemia. The proper treatment of your condition depends on its cause. Hypoglycemia is not in itself a disease or a specific diagnosis. It is a manifestation of an underlying disease, the correction of which should raise the level of your blood sugar.

The cause of your hypoglycemia at this point may already be obvious to your physician. Pregnancy, for example, or previous ulcer surgery, alcohol intake after a prolonged fast, or overtreatment with insulin are easily diagnosed without resorting to sophisticated tests. On the other hand, if the cause of your low blood sugar is not clear, you may need further testing and possibly even hospitalization.

As reviewed in Chapter 9, one of the first maneuvers will be to determine whether your blood sugar falls abnormally low in the *fasting* state. If it does, thorough and complete evaluation is mandatory, since some causes of fasting hypoglycemia can be life-threatening. Your physician may wish to consult with a specialist in endocrinology and metabolism, or a specialist in internal medicine with expertise in glucose metabolism, if necessary, to arrive at a definite diagnosis.

5. Make sure you have the disease before you take the treatment. After your doctor comes up with a specific diagnosis for your case of hypoglycemia, he or she will probably suggest a treatment. Having read this book, you now know enough about hypoglycemia to understand your doctor's explanation of what is wrong, and why his treatment should help. If you find yourself unable to comprehend his explanations, it may be that they are not founded on the facts. You have every right to a second opinion if you feel uncertain as to what to do. This might well be sought from a specialist in endocrinology and metabolism. Your doctor can refer you to one. The correct diagnosis and treatment plan should make sense to you and to the specialist.

In addition to your personal physician's knowledge of the competence of his colleagues, there are other aids available for finding a reliable specialist. The American Board of Internal Medicine conducts rigorous examinations that verify the competence of specialists in the field of endocrinology. Those who pass these examinations are known as "board-certified" endocrinologists. Your local county medical society office can provide you with the names and addresses of board-certified endocrinologists in your area. You can find the number of the office of your county medical society in the telephone book.

A publication known as the *Directory of Medical Specialists* also lists addresses of specialists of all sorts throughout the United States and includes information on board certification. While passing an exam and having a certificate do not ensure that a doctor can give quality care, they do provide evidence of a significant level of competence.

Another source of reliable referral can be the nearest medical school or teaching hospital affiliated with a medical school. You could call the office of the chief of the department of medicine and ask for the name of a well-trained specialist in the area.

In many cases, referral to a specialist is unnecessary. For example, hypoglycemia that occurs *only* after eating and never in the fasting state has few known causes. A specialist may add little to what you (having read this book) and your physician already know about the subject.

6. Avail yourself of the advantages of modern medicine. Blood glucose metabolism is an area of scientific progress and achievement. You should take advantage of it. If you live in modern America and have a transportation problem, such as a 50-mile commute to work, it would be unfortunate to be relying on a horse and buggy to get back and forth each day. Similarly, if you have a problem with low blood sugar, it would be unfortunate to be relying on a physician still wedded to the use of adrenal cortical extract.

Hypoglycemia is a biochemical matter. It is in the province of those trained in body chemistry, such as medical doctors specializing in internal medicine or endocrinology and metabolism.

While those who manipulate the spine make many people feel better, including many suspected of having low blood sugar, a *proved* case of *fasting* hypoglycemia should really be in the hands of a medical specialist. Competent chiropractors would refer cases of fasting hypoglycemia to their medical colleagues.

Likewise, those who heal through the manipulation of diet and the provision of trace elements and vitamins make many people feel better. Otherwise they wouldn't flourish as they do. Indeed, dietary modification is an important part of the treatment of several causes of hypoglycemia. Before treating your hypoglycemia, however, your physician should seek a specific diagnosis. Blood-chemistry tests—not hair clippings or personality profiles or X-rays of the spine—are necessary for the intelligent evaluation of low blood sugar.

A good medical doctor can and should provide you with all the benefits of a "holistic" or "whole-person" approach. The preventive aspects of good nutrition, exercise, and a healthy outlook are completely compatible with the intelligent use of modern methods for diagnosis and treatment of disorders causing hypoglycemia. You don't need to forsake modern medicine to find a physician who cares about you, and not just about your disease.

7. Don't insist on having hypoglycemia. Occasional patients are "bound and determined" that they have hypoglycemia even though the facts—the blood sugar measurements—refute that diagnosis. Their symptoms fit so well with the descriptions of hypoglycemia they have read, and they feel so much more comfortable having a specific diagnosis, that they latch firmly on to that one. Perhaps some of these people feel that they will be accused of being neurotic, or hypochondriac, unless they have a specific physical ailment that they can name and that accounts for their symptoms. This anxiety to be ill for the wrong reasons can divert you from getting on with what can be done to feel better.

I suspect the medical profession has created this defensiveness on the part of patients. When some doctors don't know exactly why someone is feeling sick, they may say it is either a virus, or mental, emotional, or "psychosomatic." Since doctors don't have readily available tests to prove or disprove either of these diagnoses, they put themselves in a comfortable position by ascribing your symptoms to your emotions or a virus. They also thereby leave you with little in the way of helpful treatment. In addition, implicit in the "psychosomatic" diagnosis is a hint that it's your own fault that you're sick, not the doctor's fault that he can't help you. No wonder patients feel uncomfortable with a diagnosis of a psychosomatic disorder.

Some physicians have sensed this discomfort on the part of their patients, and have responded in one of two ways: First, they have invented polite names for psychosomatic illnesses; second, they have latched on to idiopathic reactive hypoglycemia as a new catch-all diagnosis, one that could stand beside viruses and anxiety as a way of explaining symptoms to themselves and to the patient. By using it, the doctors have made themselves feel better, creating a comforting illusion that they were wise enough to diagnose the problem. This approach may also help the patient relax because the doctor knows what is going on and can treat it. Moreover, many of the treatments have been fairly harmless.

Please note that I am not saying that viruses, anxieties, and hypoglycemia do not exist. Neither am I saying that hypoglycemia is due to a virus or to anxiety. The message is that each of these three categories of disease, while authentic, has been abused at times by the medical profession, and physicians have lumped many patients into those categories on insufficient evidence. Don't let yourself be lumped into a category that doesn't apply to the facts of your case.

If being misdiagnosed as hypoglycemic and eating a "hypoglycemic diet" makes you feel well, that is fine as long as the diet is nutritionally sound. If you really have hypoglycemia, however, you had best obtain more specific diagnosis and treatment. And if you don't have hypoglycemia, it is time to start figuring out what you do have.

8. Take steps to promote your well-rounded health. Don't overconcentrate on one narrow aspect of health and disease—such as blood sugar—because you'll miss opportunities to improve your health. While your physician is searching for a specific diagnosis to account for your symptoms, there is much *you* can do to feel better. For example, you can stop smoking. This alone would do more for most people's health than a consultation with an endocrinologist, and would cost less. You can start a sensible diet and shed those excess pounds. You can start exercising, go to bed on time, cut down on coffee and alcohol. In other words, the medical profession by itself is unable to provide you with good health. You hold as many keys as your doctor does, and if you don't use them to promote a sense of well-being, there is no way he can make you whole. Moreover, medical scientists have much left to discover, and don't yet know the cause or cure of many symptoms that afflict the human race.

SUMMARY

To summarize some simple dos and don'ts for suspected victims of hypoglycemia:

1. Read Chapters 1 through 4 to understand the basic facts about the nature, symptoms, and detection of hypoglycemia.
2. See your family doctor, and discuss your symptoms with him, as previewed in Chapter 9.
3. Have your blood glucose measured during the symptoms that raise the possibility of hypoglycemia.
4. Don't insist on having hypoglycemia unless your symptoms are accompanied by abnormally low levels of blood glucose.
5. If your blood sugar is low, press for a diagnosis of *why* it is low.
6. Be sure you grasp the logic of your treatment, which should derive from a specific diagnosis of the cause of your hypoglycemia.
7. If you have hypoglycemia, take advantage of medical progress by working with a physician in the mainstream of scientific medicine.

In conclusion, although hypoglycemia has been a medical fad, it does in fact exist. Now that you understand low blood sugar, you can help your physician determine whether you really have it. If you do have hypoglycemia, you need specific diagnosis of its underlying cause as the basis for intelligent treatment.

For your reference, the final section of this book reviews words and concepts essential for an up-to-date understanding of hypoglycemia.

Glossary of Terms Related to Hypoglycemia

All terms in this chapter appear alphabetically. For the pages in previous chapters that provide further explanation of these concepts, the reader may consult the index.

ACE See **adrenal cortical extract.**

Ackee Fruit When unripe, this fruit contains a powerful poison known as hypoglycin. It blocks gluconeogenesis, and therefore causes hypoglycemia in the fasting state. After the fruit has fully ripened, the hypoglycin is no longer present; it is then fit for consumption. "Jamaican vomiting sickness" is the full-blown illness caused by eating the unripe fruit. The name derives from the vomiting that is a prominent symptom in this poisoning, and from the abundance of ackee trees in Jamaica.

Adrenal Cortical Extract Sometimes abbreviated ACE, this is an obsolete preparation made from animal adrenal glands. It is not potent enough for the treatment of adrenal-gland failure, and is not part of the intelligent treatment of any known cause of hypoglycemia.

Adrenal Glands Often called "the adrenals" for short, these glands are perched on top of your kidneys. They make several important hormones, including cortisol and epinephrine, both of which raise the level of blood glucose. Failure of the adrenal glands to make these hormones is a rare cause of hypoglycemia.

Adrenal Insufficiency Failure of the adrenal glands to make their hormones; sometimes called Addison's disease. It is a rare cause of hypoglycemia, requiring hydrocortisone or a similar product for treatment. "Adrenal cortical extract" is not an adequate treatment for this unusual condition, which would preferably be managed under the supervision of a specialist in internal medicine or endocrinology.

Adrenalin Popular term for epinephrine, a hormone made in the adrenal gland. See **epinephrine; adrenergic symptoms; beta-blockers.**

Adrenals Medical jargon for the adrenal glands.

Adrenergic Symptoms Symptoms caused by adrenalin, such as rapid heartbeat, shakiness, perspiration, and anxiety. These symptoms, explained further in Chapter 2, often occur when the blood sugar is low. Conditions other than hypoglycemia can also trigger them.

Alanine One of the amino acids. Alanine is important in glucose metabolism because it is used by the liver and kidney as a building block for the production of new glucose (gluconeogenesis).

Amino Acids These are the basic building blocks of protein. There are more than 20 different amino acids. The liver converts several amino acids, especially alanine, into glucose in the process of gluconeogenesis.

Anemia A low blood level of hemoglobin, the pigment in the blood that carries oxygen and gives blood its red color. Because anemia is a fairly common and familiar term, it is discussed in this book for purposes of analogy. Anemia is comparable to hypoglycemia in the sense that (1) its symptoms are not unique to that condition, (2) it is diagnosed by making a measurement of the amount of something in the blood (hemoglobin in the case of anemia; glucose in the case of hypoglycemia), (3) it is not in itself a disease, but is rather a manifestation of some underlying problem, and therefore (4) although it can be immediately relieved by replacing the deficient material in the bloodstream, its intelligent long-term treatment depends on identification of its underlying cause.

Anti-insulin Hormones Not an official term, but used in this book to denote hormones that have effects on blood sugar opposite those of insulin. In other words, they raise blood sugar. These hormones include glucagon, epinephrine, cortisol, and growth hormone. The medical literature often refers to them as the "counterregulatory" hormones, but "anti-insulin" should be clearer to most readers.

Beta-blockers Medical jargon for a series of drugs that interfere with certain actions of epinephrine or adrenalin. These drugs include propranolol, nadolol, atenolol, and timolol and are used in treatment of conditions as diverse as migraine headache, glaucoma, high blood pressure (hypertension), tremor, irregular heartbeat, and heart attack. Their side effects include masking the adrenergic symptoms of hypoglycemia, and impairing recovery from low blood sugar. Because they help prevent adrenergic symptoms, they have provided relief for some persons with normal blood sugar who have symptoms similar to those caused by hypoglycemia.

Carbohydrates One of the three main classes of foods essential for nutrition. The others are fats and proteins. Carbohydrates serve as fuel for energy, and also as structural components of tissues. Carbohydrates include all sugars and starches. Important dietary sources of carbohydrates include grains, potatoes, milk, fruits, and vegetables. Carbohydrates are an essential part of balanced nutrition and should not be excluded from the diet. The carbohydrate sucrose, however, can be excluded from the diet without harm as long as one takes in adequate amounts of other carbohydrates, such as occur in grains, fruits, and vegetables.

Cortisol An important hormone made in the outer layer (cortex) of the adrenal glands. Cortisol raises blood glucose by promoting gluconeogenesis, and by facilitating the breakdown of glycogen by glucagon and epinephrine. Lack of cortisol can therefore lead to low blood sugar. This lack can be treated by giving medications, such as cortisone or hydrocortisone, which act like cortisol in the body. Too much cortisol, cortisone, or hydrocortisone causes high blood sugar.

Cortisone See **cortisol; hydrocortisone.**

C-peptide A portion of the proinsulin molecule that is split off during the manufacture of insulin within the islets of Langerhans. The pancreas secretes C-peptide into the bloodstream with insulin. One C-peptide enters the bloodstream with each molecule of insulin. On the other hand, insulin injected by syringe is not accompanied by C-peptide, since the pharmaceutical companies that produce insulin purify it, removing the C-peptide fragments. Physicians can measure the C-peptide level in the bloodstream of a patient with hypoglycemia caused by too much insulin and thereby determine whether the insulin came from the pancreas or from an injection. Patients who are making themselves hypoglycemic by shots of insulin will have low C-peptide levels, whereas patients with insulinoma will have high C-peptide levels.

Dextrose See **glucose.**

Diabetes Mellitus High blood sugar—not momentarily high blood sugar, such as could be produced in anyone by giving lots of glucose by vein, but a chronically elevated level. When an elevated level of blood glucose persists over many years' time, there is often damage to nerves, eyes, and kidneys, and an increase in hardening of the arteries. These effects of chronically high blood sugar are known as the "complications of diabetes."

Diabetes mellitus is to be distinguished from diabetes insipidus. *Diabetes* refers to copious urination, as lots of water passes through the body. *Mellitus* means "sweet," whereas *insipidus* means "tasteless." Inquisitive physicians discovered long ago that some people afflicted with copious urination had urine that tasted sweet (because of its high sugar content), while others had urine that didn't taste sweet. So they divided diabetes into diabetes mellitus (in which blood and urine sugar levels are high) and diabetes insipidus (in which sugar levels are normal). Diabetes insipidus has nothing to do with blood sugar levels, and it is caused by problems entirely different from those that produce diabetes mellitus.

Diabetes mellitus, or chronically high blood sugar, can be treated basically in four ways: (1) Insulin, given by injection or stimulated from one's pancreas by drugs, lowers the level of blood glucose. (2) A reduction in food intake lessens the input of glucose into the bloodstream, and thereby lowers the resulting level of blood glucose. (3) Exercise, if there is at least some insulin present in the body, causes glucose to flow from the bloodstream into muscles, which use the glucose for energy. Since exercising muscles drain glucose from the bloodstream, the blood glucose level falls. (4) Reduction or elimination of anti-insulin influences, such as the hormones glucagon, growth hormone, epinephrine, and cortisol, lowers the blood glucose. Since infection often stimulates these hormones, the treatment of infection usually improves blood sugar in diabetes mellitus. Obesity also interferes with the action of insulin, so diabetic patients who are overweight should reduce. Other anti-insulin influences include antibodies that block the action of insulin on cells and tissues. Measures to reduce these influences allow the blood glucose to come down toward normal.

The rational treatment of high blood sugar, just as that of low blood sugar, depends on the cause of the abnormal level of blood sugar. For example, the diabetic who totally lacks insulin should have insulin shots, whereas the diabetic who is obese should go on an exercise and weight-loss program.

Digestion The breaking down of complex foods into simple molecules that can be absorbed from the intestine into the bloodstream. Protein, for example, is digested by the action of stomach acid and pancreatic enzymes into its component building blocks (amino acids), which can then be absorbed. Starch is digested into simple sugars by the action of enzymes in saliva and pancreatic juices and of other enzymes that line the walls of the intestine. Fats are similarly digested into their component parts prior to absorption into the bloodstream.

Endocrine Gland A gland that produces a hormone. Examples of endocrine glands include the adrenal glands, the pituitary gland, the thyroid gland, and the islets of Langerhans in the pancreas. The term *endocrine* distinguishes these glands from *exocrine* glands. Exocrine glands are *not* endocrine glands and do not make hormones. Instead, exocrine glands make substances that are secreted either to the outside of the body (such as the sweat glands of the skin and the milk glands of the breast) or into the gastrointestinal tract (such as saliva glands, the mucus glands of the intestine, and the portion of the pancreas that produces digestive enzymes for secretion into the intestine). The exocrine glands have ducts (tubes) that convey the material secreted either to the outside of the skin or the inside of the gastrointestinal tract. Endocrine glands, on the other hand, do *not* have ducts. Their secretions (hormones) pass through the walls of the cells that produce them and directly into the bloodstream. Because they do not have ducts, the endocrine glands used to be known as the "ductless glands."

Endocrinologist A doctor specializing in endocrinology and metabolism. Since hormones and metabolism affect every tissue in the body, a medical endocrinologist should first be trained in general internal medicine. He or she would then have specialized training in diseases having to do with hormones, the endocrine glands, and body chemistry. Conditions frequently treated by endocrinologists include abnormally high or low blood levels of glucose, calcium, cholesterol, sodium, and potassium. Their speciality also includes thyroid, pituitary, and adrenal problems, menstrual disorders, growth problems in children, puberty that comes too early or too late, excess hair growth in women, infertility, recurrent kidney stones, abnormal loss of bone mineral, and other aspects of disordered body chemistry and hormones.

Endocrinology The branch of science and medicine that deals with hormones and the endocrine glands.

Enzymes Protein molecules which control the rate of biochemical processes, such as glucose production and glycogen breakdown. Thousands of different enzymes exist, each controlling specific chemical reactions. Collectively, enzymes have been referred to as "the machinery of the cell" because they govern the chemical processes which sustain life.

Epinephrine This hormone, popularly called adrenalin, is made in the center portion of the adrenal glands. It raises blood sugar principally by promoting glycogen breakdown. It also promotes ketone production, thereby lessening glucose outflow to the tissues as the ketones provide an alternative fuel for muscles and brain to use instead of glucose.

Epinephrine, or adrenalin, causes the heart to beat forcefully and rapidly, induces sweating, and makes the hands shake. Sometimes it makes the knees shake or the entire body feel as if it were quivering inside. High levels of epinephrine also engender a sensation of anxiety and alarm. All these symptoms are called "adrenergic" because they are caused by adrenalin.

Certain drugs, known as "beta-blockers," interfere with many of the actions of adrenalin, including the recovery from hypoglycemia and the production of adrenergic symptoms.

Fasting Hypoglycemia Low blood sugar occurring when one has had nothing to eat for several hours or more. There are many causes of fasting hypoglycemia, some of them serious threats to life and health.

Fructose A chemical form of sugar, also called levulose, or fruit sugar. Fructose and glucose are both abundant in honey and many fruits. Sweeter than sucrose, fructose is used as a sweetener in the treatment of diabetes. The intestine absorbs fructose more slowly than glucose. When fructose is eaten, it goes to the liver, where it is broken down into smaller fragments. These fragments can then be used to manufacture glucose, which can be either stored as glycogen or released into the bloodstream. Because of this circuitous path from fructose to glucose, intake of fructose will not raise your blood glucose as rapidly or as much as the intake of an equal amount of glucose. Moreover, fructose does not provoke the pancreas to secrete insulin. It is therefore used in the treatment of some patients with reactive hypoglycemia.

Galactose A simple sugar that occurs naturally as a component of the complex sugar lactose (milk sugar). See **Galactosemia.**

Galactosemia A rare cause of hypoglycemia, in which the body cannot metabolize galactose properly because of an inherited lack of the necessary enzymes. Symptoms may begin very early in life, since milk contains galactose in the form of lactose, the milk sugar. The effects of this disease include hypoglycemia, cataracts, brain and liver damage, and in some cases impaired growth. Treatment consists of avoiding foods that contain galactose.

Gastrointestinal Tract See **Intestine** for explanation.

Gland An organ that secretes a substance for export. There are several different types of glands. The type of gland discussed in this book is *endocrine.* Endocrine glands secrete hormones into the bloodstream. Examples of endocrine glands include the thyroid, the pituitary, the adrenals, and the islets of Langerhans in the pancreas.

Other types of glands are *exocrine* and *paracrine.* Exocrine glands secrete substances to the outside of the body (such as the sweat glands and the milk glands) or to the inside of the gastrointestinal tract (such as the saliva glands and the acid-producing glands of the stomach and the part of the pancreas that makes digestive enzymes). Paracrine glands secrete substances that affect the function of surrounding cells, without having to pass through the bloodstream as hormones do.

Glucagon Made in the islets of Langerhans in the pancreas, glucagon is a hormone that raises the blood sugar. It does so by promoting glycogen breakdown and gluconeogenesis. Glucagon also promotes the formation of ketones. It thus provides not only glucose but also alternative energy sources to the bloodstream when the level of blood sugar is low. Triggers for glucagon secretion include low blood sugar, and protein intake.

Glucagon is thought to protect us from hypoglycemia during a meal of pure protein. Since protein stimulates insulin secretion, the intake of a pure-protein meal would cause a drop in the blood sugar except for the fact that glucagon also emerges from the pancreas in response to a protein meal and opposes the action of insulin on blood sugar.

A deficiency of glucagon has not been clearly established as a sole cause of hypoglycemia, apparently because glucagon is so much less important than insulin in the minute-to-minute regulation of blood glucose levels within the normal range. Diabetic patients taking insulin, however, are much more susceptible to severe attacks of hypoglycemia if their glucagon secretion is sluggish or absent.

Gluconeogenesis The production of new molecules of glucose within the body. This production occurs primarily in the liver, but also in the kidney during prolonged starvation. A healthy liver, healthy kidneys, the proper hormones and enzymes to control the process, and the building blocks from which glucose is made are all necessary for successful gluconeogenesis.

The building blocks used for glucose production are amino acids (liberated from muscle), glycerol (liberated from fat), and lactic acid (also from muscle). Hormones play an important part in the release of these building blocks into the bloodstream. For example, a low level of insulin allows glycerol to be liberated from fat, and amino acids to be liberated from muscle.

Failure of gluconeogenesis causes hypoglycemia in the fasting state. Once the body has stopped absorbing glucose from the intestine after a meal and has depleted its stores of glycogen it must rely on gluconeogenesis as its only remaining source of glucose. When gluconeogenesis is blocked, as by alcohol, a missing enzyme, liver disease, or lack of building blocks, hypoglycemia ensues.

Glucose The chemical form of sugar normally found in the bloodstream, necessary as an energy source for the function of the brain. Sometimes called dextrose. For explanation of other sugars, see the terms **Fructose; Lactose; Sucrose; Sugar.**

Glucose Tolerance Test This test involves the administration of a large dose of sugar followed by repeated measurements of blood glucose. It comes in two forms. In the *oral* glucose tolerance test the dose of sugar is given by mouth. In the *intravenous* glucose tolerance test it is given by vein. Neither the oral nor the intravenous glucose tolerance test is appropriate as a way to find out whether a person has hypoglycemia, for the reasons explained in Chapter 5.

Glycogen Sometimes called "animal starch," glycogen consists of many glucose molecules chained together for storage. Glycogen is present in muscles and in the liver, providing a readily available source of glucose. Muscle glycogen is consumed locally, whereas liver glycogen can liberate glucose for export into the bloodstream.

Hormones such as insulin, glucagon, and epinephrine control the manufacture and breakdown of glycogen. They do so by influencing the activity of the enzymes that chain the glucose molecules together, and then split them apart when more glucose is needed. Glycogen accumulates in the liver when too much insulin is present, or when the enzymes required for glycogen breakdown are absent. Both of these situations result in hypoglycemia, as the glucose cannot get out of its storage depot in the liver and into the bloodstream as needed.

Glycogen Breakdown The process of splitting glycogen into its component glucose molecules, which are then released into the circulation, thereby raising the blood sugar. (The formal scientific term is "glycogenolysis," which I avoided in this book out of compassion for the reader.) Glycogen breakdown is encouraged by low levels of insulin, high levels of glucagon and epinephrine, and an adequate minimal supply of cortisol. These hormones control the activity of the enzymes that break the glycogen down to glucose. Lack of the necessary enzymes and the wrong amounts of required hormones can block glycogen breakdown and lead to hypoglycemia.

Growth Hormone Secreted from the pituitary gland, growth hormone promotes growth and raises the blood sugar. Growth hormone raises the blood sugar by impairing outflow of glucose from the bloodstream into the tissues, and also by fostering gluconeogenesis. Too much growth hormone is a rare cause of diabetes mellitus (high blood sugar), and too little growth hormone is a rare cause of hypoglycemia (low blood sugar). Growth-hormone deficiency does cause hypoglycemia in children, but seldom if ever in adults unless that adult has some other additional cause of low blood sugar.

Hereditary Fructose Intolerance A rare familial condition in which the intake of fructose-containing foods produces hypoglycemia. Symptoms usually start in the first year of life when the baby begins to take artificial formula or other foods to which sucrose or fructose has been added. Common symptoms include poor feeding, failure to thrive, vomiting, apathy, and crying. Liver enlargement and eventually permanent liver damage occur if the disease is not treated. Avoidance of fructose prevents the manifestations of this disease, including hypoglycemia.

In normal persons, of course, fructose does not lower the blood glucose level at all. In fact, fructose is unique among common dietary sugars in not stimulating the pancreas to release insulin.

The exact cause of low blood sugar in hereditary fructose intolerance is not known, but appears to be an enzyme defect that interferes with input of glucose from the liver into the bloodstream.

Hormone A substance that is produced within the body and then travels through the bloodstream to other parts of the body and influences the function of cells and tissues. For example, the islets of Langerhans in the pancreas produce a hormone called insulin. Insulin enters the bloodstream, which carries it throughout the body. When insulin gets to fat tissue, it causes the fat cells to take up sugar from the bloodstream, take up fat from the bloodstream, and stop releasing fatty acids into the bloodstream. When insulin arrives in the liver, it stimulates the production of glycogen and inhibits the liberation of glucose from glycogen. There are *many* hormones in addition to insulin. Other hormones include glucagon, growth hormone, thyroid hormone, cortisol, epinephrine, thyroid hormone, estrogen, and testosterone, to name only a few. Hormones come in many different types and have a great variety of functions within the body.

Hydrocortisone A drug that is metabolized within the body to cortisol, an important adrenal hormone. Other drugs with very similar modes of action include cortisone, prednisone, and dexamethasone. All of these drugs raise the blood sugar and oppose the action of insulin in the same manner as the natural hormone cortisol. They are useful in the treatment of a variety of diseases, including adrenal insufficiency.

Hyperglycemia High blood sugar; the opposite of hypoglycemia. See **Diabetes Mellitus.**

Hypoglycemia Low blood sugar, or, more precisely, a level of blood glucose too low to support the normal function of tissues, such as the brain, which depend upon glucose for energy, or a level low enough to cause symptoms from the body's attempts to bring the blood sugar back up. See Chapters 1, 2, and 3.

Insulin A hormone, produced in the pancreas, which lowers blood glucose in several ways. First, it causes the liver to trap glucose coming into the body from the intestine and to store it as glycogen. Second, it inhibits glycogen breakdown and gluconeogenesis. Third, it promotes transfer of glucose out of the bloodstream and into the body tissues. Fourth, it inhibits the breakdown of body fat for use as fuel, promoting instead the utilization of glucose from the bloodstream.

Insulinoma A tumor of the insulin-producing cells in the pancreas. These tumors make insulin and secrete it into the bloodstream regardless of the level of blood glucose, and therefore cause hypoglycemia. Insulinoma is a rare condition. Most insulinomas are benign, or not cancerous. A few are malignant, or cancerous, which means that they can spread within the body.

Internal Medicine The branch of medicine dealing with health and diseases of adults. Internal medicine does not include surgery, obstetrics, or pediatrics; instead it concentrates on the promotion of health and the prevention, diagnosis, and nonsurgical treatment of disease in adults.

Internist A medical doctor specializing in internal medicine. Not to be confused with an "intern," who is a doctor, usually fresh out of medical school, taking a year of intensive in-hospital training. An intern could be specializing in a field other than internal medicine, such as surgery or pediatrics. An internist, on the other hand, has already completed his internship year, as well as more years of specialty training in the field of internal medicine.

Intestine A long tubular structure, sometimes called "the intestines," which runs from the stomach to the rectum. Its main purpose is to complete the digestion of food, and then to absorb into the bloodstream the useful nutrients and water while disposing of the rest as feces. It also releases hormones that stimulate the pancreas to secrete insulin and digestive enzymes. The intestine is subdivided into the small intestine and the large intestine. The small intestine is where most digestion and absorption take place. The first part of the small intestine, nearest the stomach and pancreas, is called the duodenum. The next portion, going downstream toward the rectum, is the jejunum, and then comes the ileum. The ileum attaches to the large intestine, or colon, which ends at the rectum. The mouth, esophagus ("food pipe"), stomach, intestine, rectum, and associated glands make up the so-called gastrointestinal tract.

Islets of Langerhans Named after their discoverer, these are specialized nests of cells within the pancreas that produce insulin and glucagon. Dr. Langerhans thought these clumps of cells looked like little islands within the pancreas, so he called them "islets." The islets also produce other hormones, including somatostatin.

Islet Cells Medical jargon for the cells that make up the islets of Langerhans, which are the source of insulin, glucagon, and other hormones.

Islet-cell Tumors Tumors of the cells of the islets of Langerhans. These tumors can be either benign or malignant (cancerous), and some of them secrete hormones while others do not. Those that secrete hormones, such as insulin (these islet-cell tumors are called "insulinomas") or glucagon ("glucagonomas"), usually make their presence known first by their effects on blood sugar. Insulinomas cause low blood sugar, glucagonomas the opposite.

Ketones Breakdown products of fat that are used as an energy source for muscle and brain. During starvation, fat is broken down to supply energy in the form of ketones, and the brain adapts itself to derive a greater percentage of its energy requirements from this fuel. This switch to ketones during starvation allows the body to conserve protein (essential for strength, for enzymes to control most body processes, and for the supply of amino acids for gluconeogenesis).

Disorders in which the body cannot produce ketones (such as a rare disorder called carnitine deficiency) cause fasting hypoglycemia. They do so through the accelerated outflow and utilization of blood glucose caused by the unavailability of ketones as an alternative fuel.

Ketotic Hypoglycemia of Childhood A childhood disorder in which the blood sugar falls abnormally low during fasting as gluconeogenesis fails to keep up with the normal demand for glucose. Gluconeogenesis falters because the building blocks, especially alanine, necessary for new glucose production are not released normally into the bloodstream, for reasons yet unknown. Children generally grow out of this disorder by the age of 9 years.

Kidneys Located in the back of the abdomen, these organs have several important functions. First and foremost they filter the blood, removing waste products and excess water and salt and disposing of them as urine. Second, the kidneys make hormones that are important in blood-pressure control and calcium metabolism. Third, and most important for the blood sugar, they can manufacture new glucose, especially during prolonged starvation.

When the kidneys are severely diseased, hypoglycemia occurs because of the failure of gluconeogenesis. The damaged kidneys can no longer make glucose, and the accumulation of waste products in the bloodstream interferes with other organs that also contribute to the process of gluconeogenesis.

Lactose Milk sugar, occurring naturally in the milk of humans, cows, and other mammals. One glucose molecule linked to one galactose molecule make up a molecule of lactose. Patients with hypoglycemia that is due to galactosemia must avoid the intake of lactose and other galactose-containing foods.

Leucine An amino acid that stimulates insulin secretion from the pancreas. Several other amino acids, including arginine, also stimulate insulin secretion. Leucine, however, seems to provoke a particularly powerful insulin response in certain childhood cases of diffuse overgrowth of the insulin-producing cells of the islets of Langerhans. This condition has been called "leucine sensitivity."

Liver The largest organ in the body, the liver occupies the upper right-hand part of the abdomen. The liver acts as a central clearinghouse for most of the foods coming into the body, since carbohydrates, proteins, and some fats flow directly from the intestine to the liver. In the liver many of these foods are processed, stored, and modified. The liver makes glucose, fats, and protein for export into the bloodstream, which carries these nutrients to the rest of the body. The liver breaks down many drugs, such as alcohol and chlorpropamide, that are influential in glucose metabolism. All the main hormones that regulate glucose metabolism, including growth hormone, cortisol, insulin, glucagon, and epinephrine, do so at least in part through their effects on enzymes in the liver. Severe liver disease of any cause results in fasting hypoglycemia.

Metabolism A loosely applied general term equivalent to "the chemistry of the body." Metabolism includes all the chemical reactions by which body processes occur and life is sustained. For example, the conversion of glucose to glycogen, the breakdown of glycogen to glucose, and the oxidation of glucose to produce energy, water, and carbon dioxide are all aspects of metabolism.

Molecule The smallest particle of a substance that still retains the characteristics of that substance. For example, the smallest possible particle of glucose is a single molecule of glucose. If a molecule of glucose is broken down further, the resulting fragments are atoms of hydrogen, oxygen, and carbon. Atoms are the building blocks from which molecules are made. There are about 100 types of atoms. Each type is called an element, so there are about 100 different elements. Oxygen, carbon, and hydrogen are elements. As elements combine atom by atom to form molecules, the resulting substances are called compounds. Glucose is a compound, of which the smallest possible particle is a single glucose molecule. Comparing matter to language, atoms are like individual letters, while molecules are like individual words.

Nesidioblastosis A type of diffuse overgrowth of the insulin-producing cells of the islets of Langerhans, occurring typically in childhood and causing hypoglycemia through the oversecretion of insulin.

Neuroglycopenia Lack of sufficient glucose getting to the brain, so that malfunction of the brain occurs. This is a consequence of a very low level of blood sugar.

Neuroglycopenic Symptoms Symptoms caused by lack of glucose in the brain. They may take many different forms, such as irritability, headache, confusion, blurred vision, personality change, incoordination, partial paralysis, convulsions, coma, and so forth. Identical symptoms can also result from other causes, such as lack of sufficient oxygen in the brain.

Palpitations The symptom or sensation of rapid, forceful, and/or irregular heartbeat. Adrenalin, as well as several other, unrelated factors, can cause palpitations.

Pituitary Gland The source of several important hormones, "the pituitary" is located in the head, behind the eyes and just below the brain. The brain influences its function. The pituitary secretes growth hormone, prolactin (which stimulates breast milk production), an adrenal-stimulating hormone, a thyroid-stimulating hormone, and hormones that stimulate the ovaries in women and the testicles in man to produce their sex hormones and germ cells (eggs and sperm). It also makes a hormone that influences skin pigment, and another that permits the kidneys to retain water in the body. Because the pituitary gland carries out so many crucial functions and controls through its secretions other endocrine glands with impact on metabolism throughout the body, it has been called a master control panel for many body processes.

When damaged by tumor, infection, or trauma, the pituitary may fail to secrete its hormones. In this case, depending on which hormones are missing, any of a large variety of problems may occur. Among these problems is hypoglycemia. Low blood sugar occurs because cortisol from the adrenals (which depend on the pituitary for stimulation) and growth hormone both contribute to the maintenance of normal blood sugar levels. Hypoglycemia, however, is a relatively uncommon manifestation of pituitary failure. Usually other problems caused by pituitary malfunction, such as lack of growth in children, lack of menstrual cycles in women, or sexual impotence in men, show up first.

Placebo A treatment without specific remedial value, such as a pill with no active ingredients. Placebos often do help patients feel better, however, apparently through psychological mechanisms. Recent research indicates that the release of morphinelike substances within the brain may be responsible for this "placebo effect" of feeling better after a treatment even though it does not specifically affect the disease being treated.

Proinsulin The pancreas produces this substance, and then transforms it into insulin. Proinsulin becomes insulin by the removal of a portion of the proinsulin molecule. This fragment is nicknamed the "C-peptide." Most proinsulin becomes insulin before it is secreted into the bloodstream, but some of the proinsulin reaches the bloodstream intact. Tumors that produce insulin (insulinomas) often secrete an abnormally high proportion of proinsulin into the bloodstream. The measurement of proinsulin levels in the blood is therefore helpful in diagnosing some cases of insulinoma.

Proteins One of the three main classes of foods essential for nutrition. The others are carbohydrates and fats. Proteins are composed of amino acids chained together. Dietary sources of protein include dairy products, eggs, meat, fish, poultry, and beans.

Proteins are an indispensable part of every living creature. Enzymes, which regulate body metabolism, are proteins. Locomotion is possible because some proteins, such as those in muscle, can contract. Hemoglobin, which carries the oxygen in the blood, is partly protein. The structural components of the body, including bones, cartilage, skin, and muscle, include proteins.

Some body proteins, especially those in muscle, release amino acids into the bloodstream so that the liver can convert them into glucose through the process of gluconeogenesis.

Reactive Hypoglycemia Low blood sugar that follows the intake of food.

Somatomedin A group of hormones that are formed in the liver in response to growth hormone and mediate many of the effects of growth hormone on glucose metabolism and growth. Children with a deficiency of somatomedin are short (they are called "Laron dwarfs" after the doctor who described the condition) and prone to hypoglycemia.

Somatostatin A hormone, discovered relatively recently, that occurs in locations as widely separated as the region of the brain near the pituitary gland and the islets of Langerhans in the pancreas. Its role in human metabolism is not completely understood, but it does reduce the secretion of insulin, glucagon, and growth hormone. Medical scientists hope it may someday be of use in the treatment of disorders involving the oversecretion of these hormones.

Sucrose Table sugar, composed chemically of a glucose molecule linked to a fructose molecule. Enzymes must split these two simple sugars apart before absorption into the bloodstream takes place. Sucrose is the commonly used sugar that sweetens soft drinks, baked goods, frozen desserts such as ice cream, canned fruit, jams, and candies, including chocolates. Most of the sucrose we eat comes from sugar cane and sugar beets.

Sugar A type of carbohydrate that forms crystals and dissolves in water. The familiar types of sugar taste sweet. Sugars occur in two main types—simple and complex.

Simple sugars cannot be broken down any further and still remain sugar. They are the basic building blocks for the complex sugars. The simple sugars that occur free in nature are glucose and fructose. Galactose is another important simple sugar; it occurs naturally as a component of complex sugars.

Complex sugars consist of two or more simple sugars linked together. The intestine cannot absorb these sugars until enzymes have split them into simple sugars. The most common complex sugars are sucrose (or table sugar, composed of one glucose molecule bonded to one fructose molecule), maltose (two glucose molecules linked together), and lactose (or milk sugar, composed of a glucose and a galactose molecule).

The form of sugar that circulates in the blood is glucose. Thus, when we speak of blood sugar, we are referring to glucose in the bloodstream.

Sugar Diabetes Slang term for **Diabetes Mellitus.**

Symptom Anything that a patient experiences as a departure from normal function or feeling. For example, a headache is a symptom. So are other pains, nausea, inability to think or act normally, and so forth. Sweating and pounding of the heartbeat would be symptoms in some circumstances, such as when at rest on a cool day, but would be normal in other settings, such as while running a long race.

Tumor A growth or swelling. Tumors can be benign (not cancer) or malignant (cancer). Malignant tumors spread beyond the bounds of their parent tissue, causing destruction of normal tissues as they grow.

Most of the tumors discussed in this book are unusual in that they produce hormones that affect the level of blood glucose. For example, a tumor of the pituitary gland that produces growth hormone will thereby raise the blood sugar, since this is one of the effects of that hormone. A tumor that produces insulin, or an insulin-like substance, will lower the blood sugar.

Index